Bedtime Stories for Adults

Relaxing Short Stories That Help Calm Your Mind and Ensure a Deep Sleep, Reduce Worries, Overcome Insomnia and Stress

by

Sylvia Leghorn

Disclaimer Notice

Table of Contents

Introduction

I want to thank you for reading this book, "**Bedtime Stories for Adults**".

We all have moments of stress, deep concerns, anxiety, fear, and every sort of thought and feeling that could keep us up at night.

These bedtime stories are an ideal resource for anyone trying to find some solace and for anyone trying to shut off the mind's churning thoughts, allowing you to relax and relieve stress completely.

The following bedtime meditations will help you resolve the concerns of the day and are available to help you reach a final state of relaxation and peacefulness, allowing you to fall into good sleep at night.

Each meditation is often enjoying its own, but feel free to try several in a row to reach a more profound serenity.

The best way to enjoy this series of guided meditations is to seek a relaxing and cosy place to relax in, shut out any distractions like television or telephone alerts, and prepare to go into a deeper state of relaxation, healing, and rest.

All you have to do is lie back, relax, and listen as you get carried off into the depths of your unconscious to seek out release and relief through these creative visualizations and guided journeys into relaxation. *Please enjoy!*

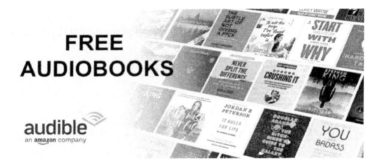

Understanding

Guided Meditation

Guided meditation is when a narrator suggests you make a specific change in your life. As the mind tends to stray where it will, many folks find it easier to focus and relax when our minds are not entirely left to their control. This type of meditation is usually guided by another person's voice - a narrator in group settings or by recordings presented on apps, podcasts, videos, CDs, etc.

How Guided Meditation Works

First, the narrator guides you to relax your body and mind, to assist you in reaching a deep meditative state before starting the journey, in your mind, to accomplish that goal.

As the brain doesn't differentiate between an imagined event and a true one, the experience you have with a guided meditation is like having an authentic experience. Due to the brain working in this way, you can change your life in extraordinary ways.

You can cause a change in your life through the practice of guided meditation. It is often because of the way the brain works. Once you experience something in life, it makes a neural pathway in your brain, and the subconscious mind will pass the information to store it for future use.

For instance, if you wanted to learn a new skill, your brain has already stored a previous experience of learning a new skill. If your experience were good, you'd be good at understanding the craft. If your experience was wrong, the likelihood is that it'll be difficult for you to get good at the new skill. Through guided meditation, you'll reprogram your brain by reaching into your subconscious and planting new and better experiences in it.

Since the brain doesn't distinguish between real experiences and imagined experiences, when you plant new experiences in your mind through meditation, your brain takes it as if you've experienced what you're imagining and makes new neural pathways to be store for future use.

Sports experts even suggest that once you try to get better at sports, and you imagine practising that sport in your mind, the muscles in your body are being activated and strengthened as a result.

Most guided meditation routines involve three sections:

•   Relaxing Meditative Session - in this first session, you'll complete an entire mind and body relaxation. It will help you succeed in reaching the meditative state required and to access your subconscious.

•   Visualization Deepener Session - in this session, we'll guide you through a gorgeous imaginary scene to strengthen your visualization skills. It will also allow you to sink deeper into the meditative state in preparation for a subsequent session.

•   Life Goal Session - This last session is where we'll guide you through a selected scene to plant a new experience in your subconscious which will produce desired outcomes in your life. It's in this session that the magic of guided meditation happens, and depending on your goal, you'll start to ascertain results in a couple of days.

Want to comprehend the science of guided meditation? Pay attention here.

Think of your mind like a video player with many videos uploaded. These videos represent a program that affects how you think, act, and behave in certain situations. These programs are installed in your brain as you have experienced them, and they become stronger whenever you have those experiences.

If you have already had an experience where you failed Math and were told that you aren't good at Math, a program in your mind is made that affects how you react whenever Math comes up. If someone ever asks you to help with a math calculation, you'll say, "I'm not good at Math" Your brain won't even attempt to attempt the analysis due to the program already installed.

The significant aspect is that the programmes were frequently created and stored in the brain and stored in your body's cells. The brain has only developed a path to coordinate your activities with external elements that interact with your body's cells.

If you stop to think about the implication of this, you'll realize that it's not our genes that determine who we are, but the pictures we create in our minds are the things that define who we are.

It's complicated to vary these programs without knowing how to access the subconscious and rewrite these programs by imagination and make new neural pathways in our mind that will communicate effectively what we want with our body's cells.

Guided meditation gives you the chance to change your subconscious by feeding it images, sounds and teaching your imagination to experience all of your senses, thereby giving your brain an experience of what looks like an authentic experience. So once you pass through a guided meditation, you give yourself an experience that makes new neural pathways that affect your whole body and prepares you for future success.

Guided Meditation for

Stress Reduction

Stress may be a modern epidemic! And you've probably heard (you can even see it in one of the previous paragraphs) about how mindfulness practice can relieve stress. But if you sit right down to training and your mind continually wanders off and thinks about the thoughts that you're trying to eradicate, you would end up increasing your stress levels! That's why guided meditations are beneficial: they mildly introduce you to the stress-relieving practice.

In general, guided meditation for stress relief, relaxation, and sleep consist of a pleasing, soothing meditation directed by a guide (an actual human or a recording) geared towards helping the listener relieve anxieties and tensions as they relax in bed or a comfortable bed chair.

Often, guided relaxation meditations involve calming sounds, comforting melodies, and the likes. These may cause listeners to imagine themselves in pleasant, peaceful environments—under a gorgeous tree by a relaxed mountain or lake, for instance, with a gradually rising sun and comforting sounds of gentle waves produced by the lake. The aim is to encourage people to unwind or relax and sleep. Some individuals discover that to enjoy their deepest sleep, meditations of this type are invaluable.

There is no telling what level we will achieve once we make use of those relaxation techniques. By learning to calm your body and mind, your physical and emotional stress and anxieties will be relieved. It leaves you feeling refreshed and more able to face the challenges the day throws at you. With persistent and consistent practice, you'll reap even more significant benefits.

How to Settle Down at Night

Sleep is precious because it's how the body heals and repairs broken tissue. The thief of sleep is Insomnia, and a myriad of reasons: anxiety often causes it. The questions would be, now we all know the diagnosis, what's the solution? How can I settle down in the dark and have at least six hours of uninterrupted sleep and awaken refreshed? Some people sleep alright but awaken tired and unsatisfied. They awaken without that spark that the majority of people that sleep well have. Why? How will I be able to settle down to sleep at night? Here are a couple of tips.

Unwind

Nothing works its magic like unwinding; that's preparing your mind to sleep. You know, the reason is a muscle and may be trained to do amazing things. One of them is teaching it to sleep—and by that, I mean preparing it to sleep before it gets to sleep time. If you prepare that you will go to sleep by a particular time, your body will be ready for it. So, conclude all of your day's activities, and start getting prepared to go to bed. Declutter, eat early, have a shower, and prepare to sleep.

Be grateful

It helps you relax if you focus your mind more on all the things you could achieve than the things you didn't. Failure has a way of making you panic, while gratitude—that feeling of contentment and peace, helps you relax. So, count your blessings before you shut your eyes; it enables you to relax.

The bed space is for sleep alone

People fall under the trap of doing other work around the space where they're mean to be sleeping. Memories work with place and time; this suggests that your brain remembers something either because you're at a particular area with specific memory landmarks or that you see things around you that will trigger that memory. If you are consistently in your sleeping space, your brain will recognize that space as your working space, and possibly that you aren't ready to sleep; it'd be a tad difficult. So, restrict your bed space for sleep alone and not for other activities.

Make sure you're in something comfortable

You do not want to be rolling around in your bed and itching; make sure that you're in something comfortable. Buy pyjamas that don't make your body itch. Make sure it's comfortable. Use clean bedspreads and duvets. If it is dirty and sandy, it is often really uncomfortable. You should make sure they are made of materials that supply you with maximum comfort.

Turn off the lights and switch on some soft sound

Soft music can ease you into your dreamland. It can function as your chauffeur into the dream world. Make sure it's not loud. Let it be a moderate and medium volume that won't wake you up, and make sure it won't interfere with your alarm if it rings. Make sure it's soft and pleasant sounding music. Then close off the lights. When it's light, your brain is active, and sleep is often challenging, so close your curtains and let there be absolute darkness. It can relax you so quickly that you nod off before you even realize it.

Organize your schedule before you sleep

We usually have a nasty habit of taking our plans and schedule to bed to plan for the next day. It is often very distracting, especially once you've got into bed and you think of something that needs to be updated or added to your list. Confirm you have all the work for the next day sorted out before you get into bed. Please ensure that your cellphones are turned off to avoid any distractions as we start to fly into our dreamland. If you would like to sleep your desire, turn off your cellphone or keep it in a different room where it won't disturb you if it rings. It's brighter and safer for you as you do not want to be woken to find out that your mom has lost her toothbrush and thinks you have it.

Get a brownout

The hormone "melatonin" is the guy responsible for your daily rhythm – put, sleeplessness and sleep. The central controller of melatonin in your body is "sunlight" or the "day and night balance," now, once you finished the day's activity, you start to ease into a relaxed mode by reducing the amount of light around you. That way, your body begins to possess a form of retirement. So, reducing the light around you can help you settle down and unwind after the day's hustle.

Use an anxiety journal

It can assist you in writing out all the tasks you've not done, all of your to-do lists for the next day, and whatever stresses you out; this may help free your mind and prepare it for a good night's sleep. You'll never unwind if your mind is carrying all the stress, worries, and anxiousness of the day; therefore, by keeping an anxiety journal, you'll set your mind free.

Reduce movement as much as you can

An excessive amount of motion in our muscles tells our brain there's still work to do. Once you reduce your movement generally and follow your routine procedure, you'll begin to settle down. Your mind would begin to be lulled into a rest mode. Another significant way to relax and unwind is to scale back your movement as much as possible.

Meditate

Meditation will put you in a relaxation mode. In a fast-paced world, reflecting the younger generations seems unimportant or overtly religious. Many of us see slowing right down to meditate as a haul. You'll easily practice meditation by getting into a comfortable position, focus on the rhythm of your breath; you could even use a breath ball to focus on your breathing rhythm. You breathe in as the ball expands and exhale when the ball contracts. Inevitably, your attention will leave the rhythm and roam to other thoughts. Once you get noticing that your mind has deviated—in a couple of seconds, a minute, five minutes—return your attention to the rhythm of your breath.

Focus on white noise

I cannot trade the squeaky sound of my old fan for love or money as the day drowns into the darkness of night; one of the ways you'll calm yourself down and unwind is by focusing on low noise. If you do not love a squeaky old fan as I do, get a sleep app and choose a sound. Keep it down so that it blends into the background. The noise from my fan, an app, or cricket can help your mind detach from the activities of the day and start to relax.

Seek help

No one knows everything; if you have any issues, contact people who can help you. Especially if you have problems with anxiety or your stress levels are very big, it's not wrong to get help from a therapist or a doctor to help with your issues. You do not want anything to affect your mind negatively. You would like to get on top of the problem and control it, so it does not affect the essential things in your life. You do not want to become depressed or experience any of the other unhealthy things that accompany it.

The bulk of your day may be crammed with different things or hustles – your mind has been alert and aware in the day; now, it's nighttime, you have to unwind and be calm for a fantastic sleeping experience intentionally. When it involves good sleep, tension is often a severe barrier; if you become frustrated when you are trying to sleep, your mind will race from one thing to another; how are you possibly going to settle down for the night?

Finding the Best Solution for Insomnia

Insomnia may be a thief of sleep; it's a situation where an individual cannot get the specified sleep. It affects sick people and other people who have bad eating and drinking habits. Statistics show that Insomnia affects over sixty million Americans yearly and may range from acute to chronic. The effect of Insomnia is often devastating and frustrating. There also are adverse consequences of starving your body of sleep like stroke, asthma, seizures, a compromised system, increased sensitivity to pain, obesity, diabetes (due to binge eating), a heart condition, high vital sign, affected sense of judgment and awareness, depression, anxiety, confusion, lack of satisfaction, and frustration. These consequences can shorten your lifetime, hurt the people you care about, and perhaps ruin your business. So how can we beat it? How do we provide it with a run of its money? Albeit Insomnia is common, there are ways to stop it from controlling you. So let's, explore them;

It all starts in the mind

The part of you that affects your sleep is your mind. Your mind is the room where all the anti-sleep terrorists launch attacks. Anxiety, stress, depression, etc., all attack the mind, and once the mind is bewildered, the body will react to what the mind is sensing. So you got to work on your mind and the way it functions. You would like to focus your energy on getting your mind in good condition. Wake up at the same time of day and sleep at the same time of day.

A routine is vital here. And it's easy to handle. Just wake up at a fixed time and sleep at a specified time; your body would automatically adapt to this routine. The body may be a routine machine; it'd fight it initially, but with time, it might suit these routines, and you'd turn on autopilot from then on.

Diet and drinking

We cannot deny that our diet, eating habits, and drinking habits affect our sleep. It's an indisputable fact, especially for those that drink a lot. Alcohol can appear as a sedative, but it'll keep you up when you don't want to be and gives you a nasty hangover. It is often pretty unhealthy. Caffeine in our bloodstream can take hours to wear out, and through that period, we'll find it difficult to sleep. The more caffeine we consume, the harder it's to eradicate them from the bloodstream. Eating late also can cause an inability to sleep. Especially if you're overfed, it'll be difficult to lie and sleep due to how uncomfortable you'd be. So it's advised to eat early and decide to sleep.

Napping could be the culprit here

I know that once in a while, you would possibly want to grab a nap and enjoy the bliss of daydreaming, but napping might disrupt your sleep routine. You'd like to sleep at a specific time and wake at a particular time, and engaging in naps can disturb that. Except napping is a component of the plan; if not, it's not advisable to nap indiscriminately. They say an excessive amount of everything isn't good, so let's watch it with the napping.

Reduce worry and anxiety

The truth is, if you're not calm, you can't sleep well. The thought and worries will awaken you. You would like to sleep, and for that to happen, you would like to do away with those thoughts. Meaning, you'll expose yourself to content and knowledge in the day, which will cause anxiety or panic. Keep your information very pure and see your heart relax.

Being in shape can shape your sleep too

Exercising has excellent benefits. It puts you in shape, gets your organs working, and clears your body of poisons. It will also help you sleep as your body will burn off excess energy and keep you exhausted but in a significant way, an honest way that your body will begin to crave relaxation. So, maybe three or four hours before sleep, have some excellent small sessions and prepare to sleep.

Maintain your daily rhythm

By this, I mean, attempt to sleep at the same time of day and wake up at the same time of day. It is often vital in beating Insomnia because it creates a pattern of sleep. There could be a temptation to sleep in during certain days – this temptation is difficult for people affected by Insomnia. By all means, maintain your sleeping time and awakening time as much as possible.

Reduce or eliminate naps in the day

As much as you'll want to, don't sleep in the afternoon; this can raise Insomnia's probability because sleeping in the afternoon might keep you awake in the Night. If you want to take a nap, it must not be anywhere near bedtime – it'll distort your internal body clock.

Stay away from stimulants

For somebody affected by Insomnia, caffeine, alcohol, and other types of stimulant is terrible for you, they're going to keep you awake, alert, and restless; so do yourself a favour and stay away from stimuli.

Regular exercises

Exercising regularly can improve your sleep experience both in duration and depth. But the downside is, exercising on the brink of your bedtime will keep you awake and alert, which should be avoided. Attempt to exercise at least 3 – 5 hours before bedtime to maximize the sleep experience.

Make your bed and the bedroom an area to sleep: eliminate other activities aside from sleeping from your bed and bedroom, if for instance, you can't rest, leave your bed and go to another room or location to sort out yourself, if it's a worry, tell yourself my bed is for sleep and not for worrying. Additionally, make it your policy to not go on your phones, tablets, and gadgets in bed. What is this going to do for you? It'll make your brain strongly associate your bed with sleep, so once you go into your room and your bed, your brain knows it's time to fall asleep – stick with this for a little while and see how it works.

Make your bed sleep worthy

It's easier to nod off in a very comfortable place with a pleasant temperature, good texture of beddings, et cetera than to nod off in an area that's disorganized, hot, and uncomfortable. Do the math! For you to possess an excellent sleep experience, make your bed and bedroom as comfortable as possible. The rationale of why you would possibly be having a rough time sleeping is because your room is uncomfortable.

Do not eat just before bedtime: once you eat, you stimulate your gastrointestinal system, the grinding and churning of your gastrointestinal system can keep you awake, so for you to eliminate this, attempt to erode at least 3 hours from your bedtime.

Additionally, to the present, you ought to drink a little bit far away from your sleep time so that you do not need to keep awakening to use the toilet; this can interrupt your sleep.

Cognitive Behavior Modification (CBT)

This therapy can help people with borderline mental disorder identify and alter core beliefs and behaviours that underlie inaccurate perceptions of themselves and problems interacting with others. CBT may help reduce various mood and anxiety symptoms and reduce the amount of suicidal or self-harming behaviours. An individual who has Insomnia should consider participating in CBT. It might put you through a lot concerning this sleep disorder.

Learn to unwind and reduce stress: this has been discussed briefly in another section of this book. But I need to add that if you have Insomnia, you ought to try as much as possible to scale back stress in the day, practice breathing in traffic, practice being calm, and maintain poise in the least times.

Does Meditation Assist You to Sleep?

Oh, the discontentment and grievance that comes with making relentless yet futile efforts to sleep. More devastatingly is the indisputable fact that it doesn't just end in a night of sleeplessness. Still, its ripple effect spills into subsequent day and cause you to start a new day miserably with sleepy and dull eyes with a terrible attitude. Well, you're not alone in this; about 35 to 50 per cent of adults in the world have Insomnia. Many adults keep complaining and whining about not having the ability to sleep, and of course, they keep trying to find solutions anywhere in their reach; some have found solutions while others keep searching. I've seen what sleeplessness does to people. So I would like to supply an efficient and unambiguous answer to Insomnia in the following lines and pages.

There is hardly anybody that has not come in contact with the word meditation before. Still, it's a thing of regret that an astonishing number of individuals don't even know what meditation is all about or how powerful meditation is. Meditation may be a very reliable technique for sleep and relaxation. Meditation is primarily seen by many of us as a thing of the mind; that only affects the mind and inner soul. But you'd be surprised to understand what proportion effect meditation has on your mind and the way that it quickly enhances the relief of the body and sleep. In meditation, different physiological modifications happen, and these modifications instigate sleep by causing several processes to occur in your body. In 2015, research results published in JAMA general medicine showed that after 49 adults were all subjected to a series of mindfulness meditation, they were ready to sleep better. He reduced their insomnia symptoms and daytime fatigue drastically. What might quickly come to mind with this meditation and sleep talks is that meditation aids sleep because meditation takes you to close up and think less, then allows you only to fall asleep. Suppose that's what you're thinking instantly; you are not wrong at all. In the real sense of it, people, especially adults, find it difficult to sleep. After all, they always harbour many thoughts that they regurgitate and chew on each minute their mind isn't actively engaged in a present or tangible matter or thing. This thought makes their body and senses all tensed up and unable to relax or sleep; on the other hand, meditation allows you to quiet your mind and rid yourself of all the disturbing thoughts that won't let you have a nice sleep. So there are chances of even falling asleep in the middle of meditation.

However, there are other reasons why meditation helps you sleep better because, you see, meditation influences several processes in your body.

- Meditation helps to decrease vital signs and consequently allows the body to relax more.
- When you engage in meditation, the parts of the brain that cause or control sleep in your body are stimulated.
- Meditation also reduces pulse, which also helps the body to relax and sleep well.
- Meditation also stimulates and increases melatonin activity; melatonin is the sleeping hormone in your body.
- It also increases serotonin which highly puts the body in its relaxation mode.

As simple and unambiguous as meditation is, it can solve your issue of Insomnia very effectively, and it's not expensive either. So why don't you tap into the facility of meditation today and be free from Insomnia?

Getting to Sleep In Five Minutes

Reduce light intensity: with all lights on, it's difficult for your brain to understand that it's bedtime. So first, turn the lights off, put the phones, laptops, and tablets away and check out to consider sleeping. DO, your brain is informed that it's time to rest. Not just that, putting away your phones, tablets, and laptops reduces the sunshine intensity; these gadgets emit blue rays that prevent sleep and heighten sleeplessness. So, by all means, keep the lights out.

Kill every sort of sound and luxuriate in the serenity that comes right before you fall asleep.

Just breathe: breathing is one of the surest ways to relax. By just living, every tension is removed, and a message is given immediately to the brain with the knowledge it is asleep.

Hence, breathing exercises are straightforward because they aren't mentally engaging. To nod off faster, you'll inhale for about 6-10 seconds, hold your breath for about 8-10 seconds, then slowly exhale, as slow as you'll, do that until you gradually nod off. It indeed works, and that I am sure it'll work for you in about five minutes.

Fantasize: this is you intentionally getting your mind far away from the physical world; letting your mind stray gets you closer to sleeping fast.

All set to sleep, but sleep seems far away from you? Try fantasizing about belongings you would like to experience. Envision a journey in adventure (do not imagine what would make you feel anxious, such as being hunted by Godzilla or maybe an anaconda and damaging your original plan of creation). Imagine attaining your specified objective and handle fulfilment.

While some people say it's not safe since it damages their feelings when they discover that every unique event you just happened was only fantasy, it certainly will make them nod faster than you had anticipated.

 The next day they wonder how fast you slept.

Pretend you're asleep: fake it till you catch on. Pretending to be asleep helps you sleep faster. Just once you can rest and can't for a few reasons, Act as if you're already sleeping; in that manner, you are feeling such as you are sleeping, and you'll discover that you will eventually fall asleep.

Remember, while pretending to be sleeping, you should concentrate on trying to catch some sleep, no matter what could also be happening around you at that point. Also, try as much as you can to exclude any conversation that may come up.

Ignore discussions and familiar sounds; I mean sounds you're sure your roommate made by a familiar sound.

While in bed, act as if you are asleep until you fall asleep sleep.

How Self-Hypnosis Works

Based on Freud's work, the human mind is often split into three different areas of consciousness: the conscious, subconscious, and unconscious. These other areas are often seen as different depths of the mind. Freud believed that the conscious mind is the shallowest part of the mind and is responsible for creating a sense of the things we are directly aware of.

The subconscious is below consciousness, a more profound level – hence it's not so easily accessible and controls how we feel or react to certain conditions or incidents, supported by what we've learned through experience in the past. It also contains and regulates our essential bodily functions, like breathing.

The unconscious is the deepest part of our mind and the most difficult to control. It can include subdued memories of traumatic events.

Hypnotism works by reaching a relaxed state whereby it's possible to sink deeper into our minds and rewrite or reprogram our subconscious.

Through physical and mental relaxation, self-hypnosis can allow people to travel around their conscious minds and introduce positive thoughts and beliefs into their unconscious. Upon 'awakening' from the hypnotic state, the new ideas and opinions in the subconscious will, in time, affect the conscious mind and may, in turn, cause changed behaviours.

Hypnotherapy isn't a 'quick fix'; such methods require persistence and consistency for the subconscious to select up and apply the new messages.

Now that you have a thought of what self-hypnosis is, does one want to be self-hypnotized?

For self-hypnosis to be effective, it's essential to approach the method with an open mind. to do this; you would like to satisfy the following conditions:

- You should be ready to be hypnotized.
- You need not be overly sceptical.
- You need not be scared of being hypnotized.
- You need not over-analyze the processes involved.

It is essential to believe why you're getting to use self-hypnosis and what messages you would like to plant deep into your subconscious. Work on some short statements that you simply are contracting to use once you reach a hypnotic state. Your comments should also pass the subsequent grade:

- Genuine and honest – you'll not achieve success in planting ideas of belongings you don't want to do or achieve into your subconscious.
- Positive – your statements should be positive.
- Simple – your comments should be straightforward and not many words.
- Some samples of personal hypnotic statements include:
- To relieve stress at work, you'll use: 'I am relaxed at work.'
- To help with an addictive habit, like smoking, you'll use: 'I don't smoke.'
- To calm your nerves before a public-speaking event, you'll choose: 'I am a confident speaker.'

Remember, these statements are messages to your subconscious – use 'I,' specialize in specific actions, and always prepare your reports as present-tense facts. Consider one or two words to start with – commit these to memory and specialize in them in your mind.

Steps to Enable Self-Hypnosis

Now before you attempt self-hypnosis, it's important to inform someone around you what you're doing. Self-hypnosis is nearly like falling asleep, so it might add up to notify the person around you that you simply are getting to take a nap. Nobody appreciates being disturbed once they try to sleep. So by telling someone, you create it less likely for you to be concerned.

- To start the method of self-hypnosis, you would like to be physically relaxed and cosy. You'll achieve this by sitting in a comfortable chair with your back straight and lying on your back while facing upward. Take deep breaths slowly. Inhale through your nose and exhale through your mouth. As you breathe, make sure that your stomach rises and falls while your chest makes a little movement. Why breathe from your abdomen? Belly breathing stimulates the vague nerve, which runs from the top-down neck, through the chest, and to the colon. It activates your relaxation response, reducing your pulse and vital sign, and lowering stress levels.

- Find an object that you can focus all of your attention on- this object should involve you looking upwards to the ceiling or the high parts of your wall.

- The next phase is to cleanse the mind of your ideas and focus on the item. It will be difficult to understand, but it takes some time to focus all of your attention on the subject.

- Now become conscious of your eyes, believe your eyelids are getting really heavy and slowly closing; now, specialize in your breathing. Continue taking deep breaths as your eyes slowly close.

- Now, use your mind's eye to see the rhythmic movements of an object - the hand of a pendulum - anything regular, slow, and steady movement. Visualize the thing swing back and forth or upward and downward in your mind's eye.

- Softly and slowly count from ten in your head, telling yourself that you simply are relaxing after each number. '10, I'm relaxing, etc.

Believe and remind yourself that once you are done counting, you'll have reached your hypnotic state.

- Now you're in your hypnotic state. It's time to specialize in those personal statements that you prepared. Specialize in each account- visualize it in your mind's eye as you repeat the words to yourself in your thoughts.

- Relax and clear your mind another time before bringing yourself out of your hypnotic state. Slowly and increasingly forcibly count up to 10. Reverse the method you used before once you counted down into your hypnotic state. Use some positive messages between each number as you count. '1, once I awake, I will be able to feel awesome... etc.

When you reach 10, you'll feel fully awake and revived! Slowly let your conscious mind become conscious of the events of the day and continue feeling refreshed.

The more you practice and practise self-hypnosis, the more successful it'll become for you, and the easier it'll get for you to succeed in the hypnotic state.

What is Mindfulness?

Do you want to clear your mind and specialize in one thing? Mindfulness looks like an easy word. It suggests that the mind is fully awake and aware of what's happening, to what you're doing, to your movements, and the space around you, which may seem ordinary, apart from the disturbing indisputable fact that we so often veer from the matter at hand. Our mind loses touch with our body, and shortly we're engaged in unavoidable thoughts about something that just happened or sweating about the longer term, which makes us anxious.

Mindfulness is the essential human ability to be fully present, conscious of where we are and what we're doing, and not excessively reactive or emotionally overpowered by what's happening around us.

Mindfulness may be a quality that each person is born with, it's not something you have to "download" from the surface, and you only need to learn how to access it.

While mindfulness is innate, it is often accessed through proven techniques, mainly seated, walking, standing, and moving meditation (it's also possible lying down but often sleep).

When you meditate, it doesn't help place all of your attention on the goods, but rather to only do the practice; there's no denying the goods or nobody would roll in it. When we're mindful, we reduce stress, improve performance, gain insight and awareness through observing our mind, and increase our attention well-being.

Mindfulness meditation gifts our time once we can put aside the judgment and set free of our natural curiosity about the workings of the mind, approaching our experience with warmth and kindness—to ourselves et al.

Mindfulness improves well-being. Increasing your capacity for mindfulness is one of the behaviours that contribute to a satisfying life. Being mindful makes it easier to understand the pleasures in life as they occur, helps you become fully immersed in activities, and creates a heightened capacity to affect adverse events. By doing so, many of us who practise conscience discover that we are less prone to find ourselves caught up in anxiety or regrets about the past for a long time, are less concerned about achievement and self-esteem and are more prepared to establish profound relationships with others.

Mindfulness improves physical health. If improved well-being isn't enough of a benefit, scientists have discovered that mindfulness techniques help improve physical fitness in a number of the way. Mindfulness can:

Help relieve stress.

Treat a heart condition.

Lower vital signs.

Reduce chronic pain.

- Improve sleep.
- Alleviate gastrointestinal difficulties.

Mindfulness improves psychological state. In recent years, psychotherapists have used mindfulness meditation as a crucial element in treating several problems, including depression, drug abuse, eating disorders, couples' conflicts, anxiety disorders, and obsessive-compulsive disorder.

Mindfulness doesn't wipe out stress or life difficulties; instead, by becoming conscious of displeasing thoughts and emotions that arise due to difficult situations, we've more alternative on the way to handle them at the instant — and a far better chance of reacting calmly and sympathetically when faced with stress or challenges. Of course, practising mindfulness doesn't mean you never get angry. In essence, instead, it allows us to be more thoughtful about how you would like to reply, whether that's calmly and sympathetically or perhaps, occasionally with measured anger.

Mindfulness Techniques

There are some ways to practice mindfulness, but any mindfulness technique's endpoint is to realize a state of lively, focused relaxation by deliberately listening to thoughts and sensations without judgment. It enables our mind to re-focus on this moment. All mindfulness techniques are a sort of meditation.

- **Basic mindfulness meditation** - Sit quietly and specialize in your natural breathing or on a word or "mantra" that you repeat silently. Allow your thoughts to come and go without judgment and return to your focus on breath or mantra. Your mantra should be something positive.

- **Loving Kindness** - rather than that specialize in the breath; this system instead focuses on the image of various people: people we all know, people we don't; people we like, people we don't. We direct well-wishes first to ourselves and then, as a ripple effect, to others, which frees us of displeasing feelings we could also be experiencing.

- **Body sensations** - Notice subtle body sensations like an itch or tingling without judgment and allow them to pass. Specialize in one part of the body at a time until you have accessed your whole body.

- **Sensory** - in this mindfulness technique, your senses inherit play. Notice sights, sounds, smells, tastes, and touches. Name them "sight," "sound," "smell," "taste," or "touch" without judgment and allow them to go.

- **Emotions** - Allow emotions to be present without judgment. Practice a gentle and relaxed naming of emotions: "joy," "anger," "frustration." Accept the presence of feelings without judgment and allow them to go.

- **Urge surfing** – Access your cravings (for addictive substances or behaviours) and allow them to pass. Notice how your body feels because the desire enters. Replace the wish for the passion for travelling away with the specific knowledge that it'll wane.

Practicing Mindfulness

Post-Meditation

Whichever technique you select to interact in, know that experiencing moments of mindfulness in meditation may be a great initiative. After reflection, while our minds will likely experience distractions throughout the day, the more our mindfulness practice is developed, the more we will catch ourselves being distracted. Therefore, the more we will bring our focus back to this moment. After all, that's the entire point of practising mindfulness meditation — to make us more mindful and less distracted throughout the day.

So how does one remember to be mindful when you're not meditating? While doing your meditation, recognize how your mind feels, then take a deliberate step to hold that feeling throughout you for the remainder of your day. You'll find it helpful to make a clear plan of what you're getting to do next — maybe take a shower or get a cup of coffee — and perform that next task with an equivalent level of awareness that you experienced while meditating. It doesn't matter what you do after meditation, as long as you search for opportunities throughout your day to acknowledge the space and mindfulness you experienced in your practice.

As you can see, we just took a cursory look at some essential principles, and that I trust they're going to be of great importance to you and boost your sleep.

So, follow me on a journey in this book. I will share with you adult relaxing short stories to calm your mind and ensure deep sleep. They will also help to reduce worries, overcome insomnia and stress.

The Secret Cabin

You have just left your car in the safe lot behind you. You walk upon the woods from the gravelled lot. As you create your way onto the trail, you stop to admire the beauty. You shut your eyes as you search through the autumn leaves. You are feeling the daylight warm your face and makes you smell the crispness of the turned leaves.

While the sunlight dances behind your eyelids, you feel calm and relaxed, able to journey through this forest of warm sunshine and mellow colour.

Opening your eyes as you lower your head back, you're taking in the richness around you altogether. Many of the trees are filled with vibrant colours, some are evergreen, and a few show their branches as their shaken off the old and can embrace the new. You haven't explored this forest before, but you're getting to meet a lover in a cosy cabin that's deep in the woods.

This small escape from our technological world is precisely what you need. Taking a deep breath, you begin to wander down the well-worn footpath. The trail is welcoming you because it had many strangers in the past. As you walk, the leaves giving a slight, satisfying crunch as your comfy hiking shoes cradle your feet. The once lush forest is in preparation for the upcoming winter. Just like your body settles for the remainder, it must prepare. As you feel your body sinking into the autumnal shifts, you notice the squirrels scurrying about, collecting their supply for their long rest. The birds have mostly headed south, and the only noise you'll hear is the slight rustle of the leaves as a crisp wind blows through.

As you retain exploring into the woods, you encounter a large pine. You stop to admire it briefly, and you're amazed by the sheer size of it. It is often the most crucial tree you've ever seen. You can't even see the very top, just lush and thick, deep green branches to the highest. You wonder how long this tree has been here. The things must have been around to experience. Perhaps this tree was only a tiny sapling when your great, great ancestors were establishing the family that might eventually cause you. Of all the cosmic events and paths of Mother Nature, one has led to you. Like many stages in your life, all of them have a beginning and an ending. Nature is pleasantly predictable as all things follow a universe, the sun rises, the sunsets, and a new day comes. You want to rest in between to maintain an extended, healthy life. He planted this seed. With nourishment, it began to grow. Despite all odds, life continues. Saplings are ready to expand into gigantic pine trees. You are feeling that slight breeze because it blows through and ruffles your hair, reminding you that you got to reach the cabin. You continue on the footpath beyond the town, closer to the still calmness of the forest. The sounds of the city and busy roads are far behind you now. A foreign memory as your body adjusts to the new sounds in the woods. Your body openly accepts the welcoming relaxation that the planet is providing.

Your eyes relax with the lovely and cosy colours surrounding you, the deep amber, the golden yellows, and the harvest orange of the leaves. You meander through the wooded land, and you notice a new sound, a pleasing sound of the faintest trickle of a babbling brook. As you travel closer to the creek, you'll see the stream flowing smooth and calm, causing the littlest of waterfalls because the water caresses the round rocks. There's a striking green moss around the creek, causing an ethereal appearance to the present mystical place. The stream, clear and meandering, feel fresh. I love it could wash away all of your troubles by being near it. Let the stream take away any thoughts that are hindering you. Toss them into the stream, and they are often washed away for an additional time. You watch your troubles slip away on the surface of the stream, and you begin to steer along beside the water.

As the stream wraps around the path, you see a small wooden bridge arching over the pathway. Weather wore but sturdy; the bridge gives a little sigh as you walk across it. Holding on to the handrail, you'll feel the heat from the sun radiating through your body. Though all this land is new for you, it oddly looks like coming home. Like the surrounding warmth you are feeling around you is familiar. It welcomes you with open arms, and you wonder what proportion longer until you'll reach the cabin, how wonderful will it be? A little up ahead you, can see a split in the path; as you are approaching, you can read the hand-carved sign pointing to the right. Nightingale's cabin is exceptionally close. Travel only a brief distance,

and you will be ready for your vacation of peace and relaxation. The dense forest starts to offer a way to 50 more enormous rocks, hinting that you have explored yourself further to the sting of the mountain. To the left, you'll see because the vegetation has thinned bent moves for mountain cliffs. You'll explore those in the future. For now, you only want to settle in.

Your pack starts to feel heavy on you. As if it's been weighing your body down with every step. Your legs long to rest, but you recognize there's not much further to travel. Up ahead on the horizon, you see the cabin. The green tin roof stands out against the autumn colours surrounding it. The welcoming, warm woods and white trim make this cabin appear cosier than its grand scale depicts. The round logs only giving way to great white framed windows.

Your tiredness turns into relief as you walk up the three short stairs to the welcoming door. Seeing a note on the door, you read that your friend has gone out briefly but will return in a while. In the meantime, you're instructed to make yourself at home. You turn the knob and open the door; as you progress through the edge, there's one sight that captivates you.

The large sightseeing windows provide a picturesque mountain overlook as you'll now see the cabin is perched near a cliff. The colourful trees, spotted with occasional evergreens, are breathtaking. You concentrate on your breathing as you look among the trees, inhaling and then slowly releasing that breath. What percentage of different colours are you able to see? Inhaling, you count 1, 2, 3. Exhalation, you trust more. Do you've discovered all colours there are to be seen in this beautiful forest that surrounds you, this welcoming home away from home?

You take off your pack and see the kitchenette is to the left, the rooms off to the right, but directly ahead of you are the welcoming windows may be a great room. You set your package on the table by the entry for now. You'll settle in your things in the future. Now it's time to rest your body. The transcendent room has a fireplace with wood and kindling able to go; you notice the slight chill in the air, so you think starting a small fire may be a good idea. By doing so, many of us who practise conscience discover that we are less prone to find ourselves caught up in anxiety or regrets about the past for a long time, are less concerned about achievement and self-esteem and are more prepared to establish profound relationships with others.

You notice the matches on a cocktail table behind you, and you use them to light this flame. When the tiny fire blossoms to life with a small roar and crackles, you'll feel the warmth drifting off it. Feeling the heat causes you to realize there's a slight coldness that has seeped in from walking through the autumn forest. You shop around the excellent room, seeing the nice and cosy colours in the cabin, reflecting people who are all around you in the woods.

There is an inviting brown leather sofa in the centre of the space, with a crimson throw. You lie on the couch and sink further into the comfort, pulling the throw around you and banishing all cold from your body.

The heat is surrounding you as you hear the slight crackle of the hearth. A light-weight rain has started outside, and you'll listen to the pitter-patter on the green tin roof as you see the cold rain falling out; you're grateful to be inside, warm and comfy, with softness snuggled all around you. As you shut your eyes again, you'll feel the nice and cosy colours comforting your senses.

The cabin is quiet, your mind is relaxed, and your body finally relaxes fully, letting your arms right down to your fingers fall asleep to sleep. Your neck and everyone down your spine sinks into the sofa, resting on the comfortable top surface.

Your legs, all the way right down to your toes, sink further down off to sleep. Your mind drifts off to relax with the rest of your body. Let it relax; nothing is holding you back. Your vacation starts now; your job is to let everything slip away as your mind embraces the nothingness that's complete peace.

The Ocean Sings

You are on a small remote island. The sand and ocean pristine, the vegetation is full and lively. Simple living may be a way of life here, and it looks like time itself passes slower. There's no hurrying about as you opt to travel for a walk on the fantastic beach. The sun is low in the sky; the air is warm and excellent. The glistening sand is soft, almost white, as your feet sink slowly and softly into the nice and cosy, welcoming sand with each step. You are allowing the heat to spread around your feet but not stick as you gracefully stroll along the water's edge. The water to your right may be a beautiful Caribbean blue, with white foam bubbles because the waves gently caress the beach.

As you slowly walk, you'll hear the ocean; seeming to swell in the great distance, but when it reaches you, it's a whisper. A remnant of the sound wave it once was. If the ocean were an individual, what things could it tell you? Wouldn't it tell you of its survival and its suffering? Of the extraordinary life it provides for many? Wouldn't it sing it in a song? Hear the ocean. Are you able to hear it sing? Is it a sweet lullaby? Is it singing ever softly? As you watch the waves dancing to the song, you yearn to feel them caress your skin. Walking just barely into the water, you think the wave crash upon your tired feet.

Feel the sand beneath you subside because the earth pulls you down. Stand still; allow the ocean to embrace you. The coolness of the water quickly passes because the wave surrounds your ankles, allowing your feet to sink just a bit further into the nice and cosy sand. While the water sways out, you are feeling your body call it back to return. It does. It always does. The water goes out; it comes back in. The ocean breathes, just like you. The water comes in; you're taking a deep breath, filling your lungs with oxygen. You exhale, the water rushes out, carrying that sweet oxygen from your head right down to your emerged toes. Hear the ocean's song because it breathes with you, swaying with the gentle sounds, settling your body down into the world. Just like the roots of a tree, you're beneath the world now while still reaching for the sky, anchored into the life-giving solid base of this planet.

You hear a giggle in the distance, instantly recognizing the tinkling sound; as a young child plays on the beach. Such pure joy and happiness pull you towards it. As you approach the kid, you provide a warm welcome. They giggle and continue in their little world of pleasure. Slightly ahead, there's a bench. You opt to take a seat for a short time and enjoy the scenery, the sun low over the ocean, the palm trees behind you swaying with the sunshine breeze. The sand is soft and warm and glistening the reflection of the sun. You lay your head back, allowing your neck to relax as you hear the sounds. The ocean is singing its song because it breathes in and out. The child giggles with pure joy and happiness. This place is paradise; it's as if there's no room for the cloudy thoughts of tomorrow and the doubts in the recesses of your mind; all of your troubles got to escape.

You feel a soft tap on your shoulder, and you open your eyes to ascertain the sweet child smiling at you. The kid hands you a container of bubbles. Without speaking any words, you recognize this child is asking you to blow the bubbles for them. You are feeling silly, twiddling with this child, but there's no harm. You open the bubbles, dip the wand, and exhale gently. A stream of iridescent bubbles spews forth. The kid giggles and dances as they fall around them. You feel yourself smile; knowing the effortless effort you set on caused somebody else such great joy may be a rewarding sensation. You repeat a couple of times, but the child's parent is looking for them. They escape abruptly; you are trying to call them back, hand them the bubbles, but they're gone.

Left alone with your thoughts and the child's play, you speak to your inner child. What does one want in life? You ask it. As your mind responds, you blow an enormous, soft bubble and watch it fall asleep. Your mind is settled making the exchange; a drop is nearly as good as a solution on this island. Anything that's on your mind makes it into the bubble. Blow it away. Regardless of how big or small, each bead is satisfying just to abandoning. Collect each and each thought you have, pouring them into this bubbling liquid. Dip in the wand, and blow all of them away. It is often some time for relaxation. Nothing stands in your way except your mind. Who controls your mind? Control each thought as you make consistent, beautiful bubbles. Watch them drift over the ocean, carrying your troubles far away from you.

Watching the bubbles disappear over the ocean, you notice the sun is now even lower in the sky. There's still no rush, nothing to hurry to, nothing to stress 58 you; be and luxuriate in. The sun is wrapped in magical, striking colours. Above, the sky is pink, turning to a warm orange and yellow glow surrounding the sun? The clouds are white up high and sinking right down to grey, the darkest of blue just above the ocean. The purple just above the horizon starts so soft near the sun and falls into the black of night. You'll see the stars beginning to awaken throughout the sky, twinkling to life because the day shifts into the night.

With the darkness settling in, you opt to make your way to your island retreat. The sand is different now. It is not warm as your feet sink into the calm, coolness of the sand, still welcoming. One consistent thing is the song of the ocean. Although it's not a whisper, it sings louder, encouraging you to experience the steady cadence, inhaling and exhaling 'as you meander your way to your home far away from home. You'll see the soft glow of the porch light, but you furthermore may see the shadow of the hammock in the yard. The hammock calls to you; you aren't able to close up the ocean's song just yet.

Nestled between two great palm trees, you climb into the hammock. As you sway, you discover your centre of balance, focusing your breathing on the faint song of the ocean. Breathing gently in, you allow your feet to rest. Exhalation, you allow your legs to sink into the sturdy net beneath you. Inhaling, your back and stomach settle, and as you exhale, they sigh into the correct position of comfort. Resting your arms comfortably, you allow the breath to continue influencing your relaxation. The frogs and insects start to return alive and sing their songs. They are doing not distract you; your music has become your reflexive action. Inhaling and exhalation are the natural progressions. You do not consider actively doing it, your body will still do that as your muscles stay relaxed and your bones settle.

You peer up through the extensive palm frond outline and see every star in the night sky. The moon may be a tiny sliver as if delivering the spotlight of the night sky to the stars, allowing them to share their beauty with you. You start to draw patterns and shapes between the stars. Does one see the bear; the person together with his bow and arrows; the queen sitting upon her throne; the swan, flying gracefully through the night? Tracing the connections between each group, does one see many lines connecting all the stars? Focus harder; check out each star.

Imagine what proportion of life and potential there are seeing this same star as you at this very moment. You're no different from the other in the big scheme, yet you're a thousand ways unique. You have such a lot inside you, but you're on top of things of it all. Every thought you have, maybe a part of you. You control where that thought is stored. If it's troublesome, blow it away in a bubble. If it's pleasant, explore it. It is often some time, your vacation, you're everything alive, and you're nothing but quiet and stillness. Allow your eyes to rest just like the remainder of your body. Allow them to be sleepy and asleep. Give the mind control of your entire body; your mind gives you peace, joy, and rejuvenation. Nourish it; enjoy the song of your mind as you drift into oblivion.

The Spirit Source

That Wednesday made Quentin decide for sure: He needed to get far away from the post office for a short time.

Quentin needs to spend quite a little bit of time outside of the building as a mailman already. On days like that, his ability to return and go only made his times inside the place worse by comparison.

Nothing, especially, might be pointed to explaining his decision to use every week of vacation days. The operations of the place were just as equivalent as usual. He was returning a vital package that the recipient hasn't shown up to receive. Thereon day, like many days, it became his problem that they weren't present to take the package. Quentin gave the returns expert the box and asked her to mark it appropriately for the upcoming delivery.

For the umpteenth time in a row, she couldn't find out the way to do that walk in the park. He couldn't help her fix this — it wasn't a part of the training he had received, so he didn't skill. After browsing this same monotony numerous times, Quentin didn't think he would be ready to continue for much longer without quitting. He filled the specified paperwork and told everyone he would see them the week after.

He didn't fill the job with pain, toil, or maybe much discomfort; what he did need to affect those repetitive errors and general boredom. He knew it wasn't the worst job by any stretch of the imagination, but he knew he couldn't work there the next day. He needed time away.

The last fifteen years had been a complete experience, if not all that exciting. He has now worked at the post office for half his life; he had started as a desk attendant in high school, and now he was transporting packages to people a day at 30-years-old. Many would still consider him young, but he didn't feel particularly young after doing an equivalent job for, therefore, lengthy.

Sometimes he felt like he was an older man already, which wasn't something he liked. He wanted to feel his age. It had been hard to do when all you saw yourself doing for the rest of your life were similar to repetitive tasks he had been doing for over a decade.

He didn't know what he was getting to do in this vacation week, but one thing was needless to say. He needed to offer himself some quiet time alone so he could believe anything.

Quentin didn't know what his goal was. He just knew that he wasn't getting to work for a little while, which time had to be spent deciding exactly why he needed it.

Driving home after work felt so different when he knew he wouldn't be returning for an extended time. The chances were overwhelming when he considered them. He had some extra money; he had a whole week to do whatever he wanted. What wouldn't it be?

Without even trying, he found himself stepping into habits despite the very fact he told himself he wanted time to think. Quentin acted like he was getting to worry the subsequent day when he got home, albeit it wouldn't be for an additional seven days. When he automatically powered on his computer and played his online strategy game, he cursed himself all the while.

It made sense that he wouldn't be ready to escape an old habit so easily. Whenever Quentin got home, he often did. He didn't even roll in the hay intentionally anymore. It had been motor memory.

When he posted his first game, he groaned and packed up the pc. He wasn't groaning because he lost; he was groaning because he was disappointed with himself. Not only that, but he was mad at the "system" for creating an environment that led to habits like this.

Quentin didn't just like the indisputable fact that his job had appropriated his life such a lot that he did an equivalent after-work activity when he had a whole week to think more deeply about his life. He didn't even need to roll in the hay at home if he didn't want to. He could splurge on plane tickets and travel.

For a flash, he thought he would start now. He closed his eyes and had too many things to concentrate on. One of them stood out: Why do I want so much noise all the time?

It was no surprise that his brain had an idea like this when he lived the way he did. Quentin practically drowned himself in noise on a continuing and day today, but he had noticed this a few times now. He was a self-aware guy, regardless of what percentage of flaws he had.

He knew what was happening with him. Quentin wasn't oblivious; that was true. He could read social cues sort of a map, and when one of his significant flaws came the way of 1 of his goals, he was considerably conscious of it.

He surrounded himself with noise because he was an audiophile— he loved taking note of music. It didn't feel right to him when there wasn't music to concentrate on, even in the background.

As he tried to think more deeply, he wondered if the critical reason for his love for music wasn't as a real connoisseur but as a man who didn't want to believe his problems. While the music was playing, he didn't need to hear himself think. His ideas about the never-ending work and his sense of deception were not necessary for him. Quentin would instead have gone home a day and mask the thoughts with music instead of affecting them. He knew it wasn't sustainable.

He had thought it had been a small goal but a unique one for him. He was getting to prepare his food for dinner, but he wouldn't hear any music while he did it. Quentin would just let whatever thoughts occurred to him occur to him as he did this.

The frozen pizza's aroma coming out of the oven seemed far more potent when it wasn't being competed against by the blaring music on his headphones. He thought it tasted better, too. In only minutes, he scarfed it down and was back to face one. Here he was alone in the writer together with his thoughts, enough money to do a lot of things, and a whole week to spend it. But he had no clue about what he was getting to do.

Quentin was gone by fifteen minutes by watching his shoes at the front entrance of the house. He saw a lot of things about it that had never occurred to him before. For one thing, the shoelaces seemed long — a lot longer than he saw them be when he wore them always. Also, their orange colour was much darker than he thought it had been.

He hadn't drunk coffee or done anything of the kind; he thought it had to be the sound deprivation that made him see the planet another way. Even without listening to his surroundings, he was noticing things happening that were different from before. He had a clearer head than he had had in a while. He couldn't believe it had been just from beginning his headphones.

Then the reconsideration stood bent him since he took off his headphones: I want a purpose.

The thought surprised him and didn't surprise him at an equivalent time. It surprised him due to the medium through which he heard yet one more apparent thought; he usually saw his mind as something under his control, but when he listened to these thoughts, it didn't desire he had them actively. He almost felt sort of a passive observer of his thoughts. It didn't startle him intrinsically, but he certainly took note of the sharing.

The question didn't surprise him because he considered that question all the time while he was working. When he drove from house to deal with delivering mail and trying to deliver packages, he often wondered if this work would be his legacy on this planet.

Like all things in his life, he didn't see it as a terrible thing, but he did feel an unmistakable feeling of dissatisfaction from the items he did a day. He could rationally expect to make ok money to retire comfortably if he kept working here. On the other hand, he would never become anything. He would occupy an equivalent level of intelligence, courage, maturity. He had an idea of how, to sum up, his feelings on the matter: this was enough, but maybe enough wasn't enough.

He felt his body moving towards the coat rack. It reminded him of when he had thoughts that felt like they happened to him rather than ones he felt like he was creating: he didn't will get his jacket; he found himself doing it. He was leaving the house.

When he stepped outside the house, the rain fell much lighter than on his way home. If he was honest with himself, he hasn't even considered the rain on his way here because he was so distracted by the tunes playing in his ears.

Being outside in the rain seemed so different when he wasn't playing music; for one thing, it had been louder than he remembered. He stepped instead small puddle and was surprised at how distinctive the sound of the splash was.

His body may have propelled him to return out here, but once he was in his car, driving through the neighbourhood, it had been clear that he had no plan for what to do. He was going to need to come up with something on his own.

Since he already ate, he didn't want any more food. But he lived in a pretty rural place, so there wasn't much he could do out here. After a bit of thinking, he thought maybe he could imitate with not having music on and doing an activity with low sensory stimulation. The route from the door to the neighbourhood was a park; he could see the stars.

Going to the park alone in the dark felt strange, but it had been something for him to do, somewhere to travel. Today probably had to be weird, he thought. He had been questioning more and more lately whether sticking together with his safe, comfortable job was the thing he should do. He would need to spend some longer with himself if he was getting to find answers.

As he took a seat at the table in the park, he became intensely conscious of how important it had been that things stayed quiet immediately. He had barely processed his thought to show off the music through the music he had been playing non-stop for years. From there, he realized that he needed to seek out a purpose. His current lifestyle and livelihood weren't enough to satisfy his deepest needs.

A Cosmic Highway of Dreams

The last night of their camping excursion dawned, and Sandra sat outside with her daughters in the cool night air.

She breathed deeply. The scent of recent rain was sweet.

Nearby, the lake waves reflected the last rays of the setting sun into a golden sheen.

Everything felt washed clean and refreshed. Evergreen trees towered over the campsites, giving off the tangy aroma of pine sap.

A few birds still hooted and chirped in the trees, but one by one, they were dropping off into silence, leaving the crackling and popping fire to mingle with the soft lake sounds.

Sandra sat in a camping chair by the hearth, holding her youngest to her chest.

Kirsty sat in the chair beside her, hugging a blanket around herself. The orange firelight danced upon their features. Stars appeared in the sky overhead; white gems beset a blue tapestry.

Sandra craned her head back to seem up at them, and Kirsty followed suit.

Some stars shone brighter than others did, some were steady, and a few flickered rapidly. The view was enchanting. At last, Kirsty spoke.

"Mommy, does one ever wonder what's out there?"

"All the time, sweetie; I dream of it quite a lot. I wanted to be an astronaut once I was your age. I still think it'd be amazing to travel out there and explore someday."

"I want to be an astronaut, Mommy! Could I?"

"Baby, we've always told you to follow your dreams. If you would like to be an astronaut and see the stars, then you should do it!"

"But what if I would like to find out what the stars dream of, Mom? Does one think the stars and planets dream?"

Sandra smiled. "Well, then I suppose you'd be an artist. Poets, painters, writers, papermakers, they've all been inspired sometimes by the view from down here. Back then, I used to paint when I was a child, too. I used to know the trick to creating the paintings come to life!"

"Aww, I'll bet you'll still roll in the hay, Mommy! Just like your book!"

At that, Sandra grinned knowingly. "You mean this book, dear? This one right here?"

She lifted the heavy book and opened it to at least one of the last chapters.

"You asked what it had been wished to become a dreamer of the stars. Well, let me show you a small piece of that place. It's pretty amazing...."

The picture that graced the page was a galaxy spinning in a milky torrent of stars.

Beyond it, one could see vast nebulas and cosmic pathways resulting in the ineffable mysteries of the universe.

But the stars shone so brightly that for a flash before Sandra turned the page, night turned today in the endless night of space itself.

Kirsty gasped; then, her mother turned the page.

* * *

Jaina leaned her head against the window as the miles rolled past.

Back through the desert, where things were open and quiet, back home to the town.

She would be glad to be home, but it had been hard to leave such beauty behind.

As she searched, she saw one particular star twinkle ever brighter.

It appeared to beckon her gaze and her flight of fancy.

She wondered at its impossibly long life and its valuable distance from her.

What had it seen in many years, far-out there in space?

Jaina imagined that even stars had dreams, or even the whole universe itself was a dream to them.

After all, their perspective was so different from hers down on Earth.

She was wondering what she wanted to gaze at from this height as her eyelids began to shut, soothed by the soft sweetness of the mobile automobile.

When Jaina opened her eyes, she found that she was floating alone in the dark. No, not in the night! A lightweight shone in her face.

It took her eyes a second to adjust.

She realized that she was looking up at the half-shadowed face of the moon, but it had been so close! It filled nearly her whole field of vision.

She could almost reach out and touch it.

Jaina turned and saw below her the world altogether its glory: blue and green, white swirling clouds making pleasant shapes she recognized as birds, mice, flowers, and more.

Jaina just floated, breathlessly awed by sight.

She had never realized how magnificent the planet was, so vast in its infinite varieties and mysteries.

What an area to call home!

She could even hear its song from here, a grand symphony formed by the littlest organism to the most critical mountain in unison. Nothing could compare.

She sang another song to her.

It was the moon, a sweet note of admiration for the world that was its home also.

Jaina floated toward the moon and landed upon its surface.

It spoke to her in a voice that was both young and old, lilting and yet soothing.

"Hello, baby! You've traveled far tonight. I'm happy that you can listen to me singing to you, my greatest love."

Jaina beamed proudly, "Yes, I can! I've never seen the moon or the planet like this before. I'm very happy to have gotten the opportunity to experience it. Is this what it's like for you all the time?"

The moon glowed happily. "The view changes depending on where I am, which is why I circle the entire world. I want to listen to everything and everybody."

"Of course!" Jaina sprang lightly up, floating far above the surface of the moon. "I do, too. It's why I came out this far tonight. I actually want to see what it's like outside of what I know."

"Then you'll get to go very far tonight, little one! Let my gravity assist you along, and remember to mention goodnight once you come to this manner again."

And the moon exerted her gravity, propelling Jaina in a wide arc around her white surface.

Jaina laughed and cheered, feeling like she was trapped in a sudden gust call at an area where no air existed. She waved farewell to the moon as she sailed away.

A giant Mars greeted her with a bombastic song, like a whole orchestra of crashing cymbals and bellowing tubas.

Vast mountains and deep valleys scrawled across its surface gave the impression of a starkly rising and falling melody.

Craters pocked the surface, and in all, dancing lights of a weird colour, always in some pattern.

Waves and snowflake-like information, rippling circles, and stranger shapes appeared.

The dreams of Mars itself met with those of the people on Earth looking outward at Mars, and the result was an aurora-like luminescence that blanketed Mars. Thrilled, Jaina flew onward.

Far ahead, asteroids lay across her field of vision like dark flowers upon a starry black lawn.

Jaina swam freely through the open space to them, growing larger with each passing second.

There were minor asteroids and medium-sized ones, and ones so huge they were like buildings floating in nothingness.

Some spun inconsistent with their inertia, some floated motionlessly, and still, others turned this manner which.

Jaina landed upon one and noticed that she wasn't alone.

Little sprites danced merrily between pieces of asteroids, disappearing into one of the various holes in their porous surfaces only to emerge again with a cackle and a flash.

Jaina tried to follow them, but they were too swift for her, ever urging her on with their laughter and frolicking.

Jaina leapt after one, and it vanished in a puff, but she sailed into the tunnel into the asteroid.

Metals or gleaming crystals sparkled as she flew through a tunnel that rang with voices of fairies and capricious spirits of space and time.

Light-filled the tunnel sort of a sudden sun, but she found that she had only come to the start when she reached the other side.

The laughter of the fairies greeted her from the tunnel.

Jaina laughed successively. Their names weren't malicious, just tricky.

"Okay, keep your secrets! I feel I'm too big to suit, anyway!"

"Size is extremely relative here," said one of the spirits, appearing sort of a miniature ghostly star wreathed in cloud.

In one moment, it had been small as a baseball, and when Jaina blinked for that instant, the spirit seemed inconceivably vast because of the Sun.

"In the dreams of the universe, 'big' or 'small' is meaningless. You're as important because of the biggest asteroid, the littlest Sun. The galaxy couldn't exist without you, and you couldn't exist without the galaxy!"

Jaina's eyes grew wide. "Oooh, I feel I don't quite understand, but I would like to!"

"Then journey further; all that beckons you."

Jaina thanked the spirit, and she drifted further still, past the belt.

As soon as she crossed that border, the music of the cosmos changed.

It became loftier, more harmonic, and resonant in a way that reached into her deepest thoughts.

She closed her eyes and listened, content to be merely a fraction of the spheres' music for the moment, an eternity.

When she opened her eyes again, she found that she had drifted almost a giant planet, an excellent swirling mass of browns and reds and cream colours.

It turned to her, and she found that the planet was chatting with her.

Its voice was slow and sonorous, and it sounded just like the quiet rush of an ocean wave.

"Welcome, traveler! What brings you out so far?"

Jaina grinned in pure pleasure. "Why, just seeing what the dreams above the clouds are like!"

Jupiter laughed with a sound that rang across the whole system.

"Would you wish to ascertain what I see? Inherit my eye, and I will show you the items that even I dream about." Excited beyond measure, Jaina flew toward the Earth. "Yes, please! I would like to see!"

As she dove into the good eye, there became a perfect rainstorm surrounding her; She made only the rain from soft light.

Winds swirled about her in a choir older than humanity itself, welcoming her, buoying her with their sweet serenade. Then the swirling clouds broke, and she saw with the planet's great eye.

At one point, She cast her gaze beyond the universe with its vast frozen rings and delicate colours, beyond the planets of the system.

She looked at the distant stars, which burned with a halo of colours, serpentine "sun dogs" coiling gracefully around them, and the myriad kaleidoscope shapes that appeared in their fiery surfaces.

Each one was a lens for the dreams of foreign places, shining a lightweight into the gorgeous expanse of space.

Her gaze swung again, and she saw a vast maroon cloud unfolding.

It seemed like an enormous bird unfurling its wings, dotted with stars like diamonds studding its feathers.

Its great fiery plume slowly expanded, the entire nebula growing like an eagle spreading its wings for the flight across the vastness of the cosmos.

Points of brilliant light appeared around it in great reddish-white flashes, and in each, one was born a new world of dreams.

The birdlike nebula opened its beak and uttered a cry of creation, and from its throat flowed the things of which She made worlds.

Dust, gases, and matter flowed forth in flood so titanic it might blanket a world, spiralling together, a burning ember at its heart.

More joined the cosmic deluge and more still, and in the heart of it all, a star was born from the very dreams of the universe.

The bird-nebula spread its wings further and flew from one end of space to the other, trailing pure magic from its branches.

Comets and belts of stars and spinning rings floated outward from its wake, each happening to hunt yet more places to manifest celestial phenomena.

Jaina in Jupiter's eye blinked, then it looked further still, watching a star in its final brilliant moments before it burst.

Impossibly bright, it's light-filled the firmament. Every beam carries the needs of everyone who stared at a star and wanted to spread over the cosmos from Dreamtime.

New paths were born for those who dreamed of succeeding in the foremost far-flung of destinations, forged by the sunshine of the dying star.

Even its magnificent ending created a new life for itself and others by filling the universe with newfound hope and inspiration.

Beyond the supernova lay a band of comparable stars suspended in white mist. The entire Milky Way galaxy stretched before her.

Its beating heart was a bright white focus on which the whole Dreamtime world spiralled, all sharing the space and time.

For here, there have been no barriers between time and thought, spirit and space, dream and cosmic law.

Nebulae unfolded in silent compositions that told of the birth of entire worlds.

Stars emerged from the ether and grew into cosmic forges so hot that to strike upon them was to shape solar systems.

The majesty she witnessed expanding across the boundless universe was enough to touch Jaina's imagination forever.

She had never dreamed of anything which prepared her for the universe's grandeur and power of this magnitude.

She swam in a vision of pure bliss borne upon the very spirit of the cosmos and felt its irresistible pull.

Excellent blue stars glimmered in the clouds of reddish-white dust.

Planets swam through the ocean of space, caught in the tides cast by the stars.

Comets soared through this like great travellers exploring worlds unknown.

The universal music reached from the very highest to the smallest, leaving nothing untouched by its harmonies.

Light flowed across the known and unknown, hemmed by the dark of open space, a grand vision of eternity.

The most potent possibilities clashed with the slightest bit of impossibility to make dreams and visions happen.

A star shone in the heavens for each raindrop that received an ocean and delivered to light yet one more facet of this incalculable grandness.

Jaina slept, entirely enthralled by the visions of all that was and everyone that might at some point exist and the way it sang from the very instruments of creation.

She felt her small part therein primordial music, and she knew peace, oneness with the universe.

For only in a dream could someone know what it truly meant to be a part of it all, a wanderer in a place so incredible that it defied pure understanding, and yet never alone on the journey?

Every star in the universe shone its fall upon her, and successively, her every dream fed them.

Every time she saw a star twinkle in the sky from that day forth, Jaina knew.

The stars were dreaming, too.

The Secret Guide

You are alone in your bed or your space of comfort.

You are here to rest and relax.

There is nothing left to do now but sink into the covers, melt into the mattress, and find relief in your body after a long day.

You are here to reach total serenity, peace of mind, and relaxation.

If there is anything you would like to do to get into the most comfortable resting position, do so now

Take a moment to honour your body.

Find your stillness and your centre.

Let go of any judgments you have about your body or the way it feels.

Notice the areas holding onto something or that have tension, and let it all effuse once you exhale. Your body can begin to rest.

There's merely silent space behind all the layers of your day, job, relationships, responsibilities, or deadlines.

In this bedtime story, you're getting to find a personal guide that will take you to the present place of quiet and release so that you'll find a more profound comfort from within you.

You hold the key to your relief, and this guided meditation and bedtime visualization will take you there, one step at a time.

Your breath should start to become long. And slow. And steady.

Let it flow naturally.

Don't overthink your breathing.

Just allow it to move you more deeply into your relaxed state of mind and body.

Your physical self has been at work all day.

Even if you weren't travelling all that much, if you had to take a seat down at your desk or work from a seated position somewhere, your whole body has still worked hard.

Your mind has been hard at work.

You are always thinking, weighing and calculating, observing, listening, processing.

You have all of the energy of thought radiating from your brain and your body.

Now, you'll begin to let your energy flow in longer, thicker waves.

You don't have to be in a conservative state.

You are now liberal to sink into a state of total relaxation.

Help your body feel softer and more elastic with each inhale of breath and every exhale of tension or any quiet thoughts or ideas that keep circling.

Breathe it all out and are available to an area of peace of mind and body.

You are now in a more relaxed state of energy, and you'll fall even deeper into your unconsciousness.

You can take a journey farther than you have ever travelled before.

You can discover your highest state of relief, your most sacred level of self-healing, finding your balance with every breath as you transcend space, time, and the material world.

Begin to ascertain in your mind a bright light at the top of an extended tunnel.

The tunnel may be a part of your mind that takes you into a deeper layer of your consciousness.

You can float through the tunnel, same as s seed on the wind, going closer to the sunshine at the top, feeling yourself soften, and welcome the spiral of sun that opens before you.

The tunnel is widening as you come fully into the sunshine.

Feel it surround you, almost blinding you from what lies on the other side.

The light is so bright that it fills your whole being, penetrating your skin and filling you with healing warmth and love.

You can feel it with every breath you inhale, the sunshine filling your lungs and circulating through your body.

As you exhale now, you'll feel the brightness of the sunshine normalize, opening your sight to ascertain an excellent open meadow covered in soft green grass and flowers dancing on a gentle breeze.

The air around you is crisp, clear, clean, and calm, but your body remains warm, safe, and protected.

You can see a good range of snow-capped mountains surrounding the meadow.

It is bright and open, filled with possibilities.

You are here in this space, an area of your deeper mind.

You are liberal to explore this land, this range, this secret world.

You feel an urge to explore in several directions, and you aren't quite sure where to start.

There are many potential paths to explore, some ways you'll attend, find your most profound calm and relaxation.

If only you had a guide, a guide that would point you in the right direction, a principle that might hold you shut and provides you everything you would like to explore this place and guide you to your serenity.

As you ponder this, you feel an itch in your palms.

Lifting your hands, you notice that there are markings on your palms.

The markings are beginning to add up.

A guide is imprinted on your palms.

It shows you exactly where you would like to travel.

Your healing path is usually in your hands, and everyone you have to do is trust yourself that you already know where you would like to travel to seek out inner harmony and peace.

The guide on your hands is showing you a path to steer.

You search at the mountains and the meadow, and you discover the direction your hands are pointing you toward. Follow the arrows of your inner mind.

Follow the way you're showing yourself to travel.

Walk-in that direction, noticing your place and how it feels to possess awareness in your deeper mind.

Inhale deeply and let loose an extended, slow breath.

Let your body remain relaxed, peaceful, and serene as your mind travels to those inner pathways.

Perhaps a fog thickens on your path, or even there's a gentle river flowing across your path.

Let your imagination go free.

If you're uncertain of where to travel, look down at the guide on your hands for guidance.

Trust your intuition to point out the trail.

As you still breathe and follow your secret guide forward, let yourself begin to hunt even further down into your subconscious.

The landscape, the dreamscape, the planet of your mind can become anything you would like it to be.

Where is it leading you?

What is happening on your path as you follow the critical guide of your soul and your mind?

Is it still comforting and pleasant?

Do you desire your guide has taken you on a darker road, a more shadowy path?

Are you continuing to follow in the guide of yourself to seek out where to go?

If you observed that you're getting off the trail or feeling like you are leading yourself into dark territory, that's okay.

At this point, you need to travel to heal your deeper self and your deeper mind.

If you would like to get back on a lighter path, you'll take a couple of soothing breaths in and out and let the sun begin and beam bright, warm, healing light onto the shadows of your mind.

Let the guide still show you the way you would like to travel.

Underneath the challenges of your journey lies the solution to where your inner harmony lives and breathes.

Somewhere the guide of your consciousness is the answer to how to heal yourself on the deepest level.

Your secret guide is usually working with you to assist you to discover your path.

Now, look down at the guide in your hands.

Look to find out that in this holy wilderness, in your mind, there is an "X", which is the highest point of your search.

Do you see it?

How are you getting to get there?

How will the trail take you to the 'X' on the guide?

Looking around, are you able to see where you would like to go?

Can you sense where that X is inside this place?

Go there. Seek it out.

Find the x in your mind's land and your soul and subconscious, the palm of your hand.

Perhaps it's a straightforward path.

Perhaps it's winding and bending.

Maybe you would like to climb over a couple of obstacles here and there, or perhaps you encounter a challenge along the road. Keep going.

When unsure, check out the guide on your hand.

Let it lead you to the X that marks the spot (take several moments to look for it).

You are now around the spot where your final destination is laid.

You have found the bottom where the 'X' is painted or etched on the world or a tree.

Perhaps it's carved in the mountainside rocks, or it might be less obvious and more sort of a feeling that you know that this is often the place.

What does this place look like?

How does it feel to be here?

How long did it take you to seek out it?

Inhale deeply, taking an extended soothing breath of air into your body.

Hold it for a flash and then exhale slowly and steadily, letting the air leave you.

And inhale again, filling yourself with the sensation of discovery, the sense of finding the spot on your guide.

Exhale slowly, going deeper into your mind, deeper into your fullness and relaxed state.

Here is where your healing can begin, once you release all of the extra spaces outside of you, once you hunt for your 'X' on your inner guide while it guides you into the deepest points of growth and transformation, the most profound moments of total relaxation and relief.

Here is where you'll release judgment and

critique. 97

Here is where you'll enlist your power to resolve the most challenging moments and the most significant challenges.

Let your body sink into this space.

Let your heart resolve any issues so that you fall asleep.

Your mind is made of thoughts and beliefs, attitudes, and emotions.

Your mind is additionally made from spirit, your spirit—the vital force energy that provides you with the critical guide of your inner journey.

Your spirit aligns you with your purpose and the right path for you, directing you in a new direction a day along the way.

All you have to do is locate your focus and follow the guide to where your 'X' marks the spot.

This guide has led you to an area of total peace and inner harmony.

You are here to rest, sleep, and dream.

You are here to fall deeply into serenity and balance.

In the space deep in your subconscious, you now see a door.

This door is familiar to you, and you recognize that it'll lead you back home, back to the safety of your warm bed, back to your whole body and mind.

When you rehearse this door, all you have to do is rest.

All you have to do is sleep.

All you have to do is to dream of where your secret guide will lead you next.

Walkthrough the door sinks deeply into your mattress or cushions go deeply into the dream world until the following guide leads you to where you would like to be.

The Pixie with a Dream

If you closed your eyes long enough, you'd see the kitchen and the ball of a dough Naomi the fairy had tried to make. Close your eyes, and you'll see the messy flour-crammed desks, her perfect buttery-ruined pink dress, and bright red hair that has just enough of the greasy mess to fit her already chaotic. The kitchen was painted yellow, a bright honey yellow, which made you want to drink tea a day and look at the gardens from the window.

She stared at the blubbery mixture ahead of her and frowned; another mistake once more, she took a small portion in her hands to make sure, and it felt even worse than it looked.

She shook her head; Mother was getting to be angry again. She hated it when she made these mistakes and today was the pixie baking spree.

Each pixie family was allowed to bring the food made by the eldest daughter and present it at the fair, everyone would have a taste, and mothers would brag about how smart, intelligent, and quick-witted their daughters were.

She checked out the clock, Mother would be back from the bakery soon, and she wouldn't be happy about any of this. Was there any way to remedy this mess? What proportion of lousy luck could one person have because it seemed Naomi didn't seem to possess a scarcity of any? If only she were an honest cook like Betsy, the gorgeous pixie nearby, who was also the best and proudest snob of all times, never will there be a word in greeting, always together with her head in a cloud of arrogance. Betsy was beautiful, intelligent, and honest, and Mother would never let her hear the top of it. If only she could bake like Betsy, maybe Mother would let her be.

****

The Baking spree was fully swung, and from one table to another, mothers conversed proudly about their children's expertise. Naomi stood at the rear to avoid her Mother's sharp and biting comments and the assessing look other mothers gave her once they acknowledged that she had not made a thing.

"Don't worry Sandy! I know you tried; you only didn't catch on right this time", Lily said together with her beautiful smile. If you let your mind's eyes focus, you'll see Lily clear as day; all you have to do is to relax and follow my words. She had beautiful golden hair that makes curly waves from the top of her head to her waist. She had a shy smile but could illuminate an entire room when it had been released, and she had gentle green eyes that gave you the definition of kindness. Are you able to see Lily? You'll give her the dress you would like, but my Lily wore a green dress, a colour that made her eyes glow even more and made you would like to follow her all around the globe.

Lily put a couple of her food pieces on a tray and put them on Naomi's table.

"No Lily, you should not do that; it might deduct from your diligence, you worked hard to bake all this and you ought to show it off, don't dim your day due to me", Sandy said, already pushing back the tray.

"Enough Sandy! If you think that I'll glow while my friend doesn't have one baked good to her name, then you do not know the meaning of friendship. She continued bending in to pinch the cheeks of Sandy, "I even have an excessive lot on my tray," he remarked, "you are offending me." Your Mother will no longer distress you once she sees that you have things to show." It is fantastic to comprehend.

"Thank you," Sandy said, feeling emotions of gratitude choking her. "That's what friends do", Lily whispered, and the pixie Baking spree clothed to be a wonder. From scones to pies, cakes, cookies, frostings of varied kinds, and toppings that might make your tongue water. Are you able to see the table? It's delicious.

And Naomi's Mother could hold her head high and claim her daughter had baked a wonder. What a case she was, but one less screaming night for Naomi to enjoy.

****

Today He had announced the science fair in the pixie world. Many fairies were excited to go!

"Nonsense, only the plebs would attend such nonsense!" Mother said together with her air of authority, and each of the other pixie mothers nodded in agreement.

"No child of mine would darken the gates of that comical event. How dare they think we might lower ourselves to combine with such dirty things as grease and machinery? It might be a nightmare to tinker with those things, how they'll ruin your hair and ruin your clothes", Mrs Buttercup said, pinching her nose in disgust.

"You won't be ready to get obviate those stains for years to come!"

"Indeed", all the ladies nodded in agreement, and Naomi felt her heart drop. It was a disaster.

She found herself running through the green fields to Lily's house.

"I hate being there in that house!" were the first words out of Naomi's mouth the minute she barged into Lily's room. Lily looked at her, confused, and dropped the cookbook she had been reading.

"What's the problem?" She asked, looking around like she could catch the explanation for Naomi's lousy mood and melt it to a pulp together with her glowing green eyes.

"No one ever cares what I want! And now they will not let me attend the science fair!" Naomi said, falling on Lily's bed as she bawled her eyes out.

"Oh, Sandy... I'm so sorry". Sandy cried for hours before she finally fell asleep, and when she awakened, Lily had just the answer to her problem.

"I know what we're getting to do," Lily said excitedly. Naomi rubbed the sleep from her eyes; her beautiful red hair was ruffled and looked like a robin's nest. She tried to smooth it down but gave up when it simply wouldn't obey her.

"What?" She asked Lily.

"We'll have an interview together with your mum!"

"Are you crazy? My Mother would have a fit if she knew I used to be curious about the science fair and you'll just imagine what she would say if he heard I had plans to travel."

"And there lies your problem, Sandy. You'll hide your dreams, you'll bury them but if you do not fight for them, nobody else will do this for you and that is a fact of life," Lily said with a knowing passion in her eyes. "But I just want to travel to the science fair, does there need to be a war about it? Can't I just do what I want? Why does life need to be this way?" Naomi said, standing up and pacing the space.

"Sandy, you'll either mope about the choices life gives you; otherwise, you can get up and make the best of it, then far Sandy, you've simply been moping, and honestly, life doesn't work that way. Our tears won't suddenly make things happen and our complaints under our breath won't move the planet. it's our actions that give us the life we want!" Lily said, and every one trace of her mischievous smile was gone. It was a fierce pixie able to get her friend the insight she needed.

"How does one know of these things, Lily? It isn't like you've faced any of these", Sandy said, scoffing.

"You'll be shocked," she said with a sad smile, and thereupon, she came to take a seat beside Sandy.

"I'm the best seamstress in the whole of pixieland; wonder how that came about?" Lily asked.

"Your parents allow you to pursue your dream, unlike mine", Sandy said dryly.

"No... I didn't hand over my dreams and that I was able to fight for them. I didn't say anything behind closed doors and pretended to be happier than them. I told my parents my passion and kept on pushing until I got what I always dreamed of: my very own sewing set and, therefore, permission to travel after my dreams. You'll mutter all you would like Sandy, but if you do not tell your Mother, really tell her, she is going to never skills much you would like this"

****

Naomi told her that there was no lily to inspire her; she was crazy when Naomi informed her. "...I raised you better than this... I..."

The ranting had been going for hours, and Sandy was able to hand over and apologize about the entire thing, but Lily's voice kept nagging her.

"Mum", she finally spoke up, "I've... I've always wanted to do this. I've done all you asked me to do, give me this one chance to do what I would like for a change. I want to make my machine and know I made it with my hands and have the entire world see it. All I would like is to..." she stopped when she saw her Mother's shocked expression.

"What?" Sandy asked, looking around for what had caused her Mother's placid colour.

"I've just never heard you speak with such a lot of passion before... it's different, it's...."

"So, will you let me go?"

Mother frowned, "I'll believe it!" And thereupon, she stormed to her room.

The following day, when Mother awakened, she announced that dashed all hope Naomi had envisioned.

"To attend your science fair, you should make all the things on this list and if I see that they're satisfactory, I just might allow you to go. I'm the best baker in the pixie world, no daughter of mine should be useless when it comes to baking!" She huffed and closed the door behind her, and Naomi stared at the list in her hands.

****

Naomi hurried to Lily's house looking very troubled, holding her Mother's list in her hands. Then she told Lily all her Mother had said.

"Can't you see? It's perfect!" Lily said

"What's perfect about this? I'm not a baker; I'm a scientist. I do not want to do this!" Naomi answered, looking defeated.

"Naomi, get your head out of the dumps and concentrate on the chance before you!"

"But I do not have the skills to bake!" said Naomi.

"But you'll learn". Lily shot back

"What if I do not want to?"

Lily frowned at her words.

"Sandy, simply because we've dreams doesn't suggest that we should always be bad at everything else. Dreams give us the thrill but those other activities teach us discipline. And a disciplined mind can do wonders with a dream. We put ourselves in a box once we don't explore as many things as possible. Simply because you're keen on science doesn't suggest you cannot be good at baking. We're fairies Sandy; multi-tasking is in us. Don't throw away your capabilities; you'll be good at numerous things, not only one. Come on?"

Sandy gave her a sceptical look, but She had planted the seed. ******

The kitchen was a delight to behold. After weeks of practice, Sandy was baking the most delicious desserts she had ever made, and there was no way Mother 109 could say no. Now, if only she knew how to make the chocolate elf bagel, she had never seen anyone except Betsy make it, and she was sure Betsy wouldn't dream of teaching her.

"What are we getting to do?" Lily asked.

"I enjoyed baking and it is so much fun. I cannot believe how much I deceived myself when I was concentrating on being good at one thing: only being a scientist," she picked up a cupcake and took a bite. "This taught me that I can be hooked on something and still enjoy doing other things. I simply do not have to place myself in a box. Many thanks, Lily!" the two girls hugged, and a mild knock sounded at the door.

Can you guess who it was?

Betsy! And she was holding a chocolate elf bagel!

****

The last two hours saw Betsy teaching Sandy how to make a chocolate elf bagel, and now Sandy had finally gotten the hang of it.

"Thank you", Sandy whispered, embarrassed at how wrong she had been about Betsy; the lady was gentle to at fault, and the only reason her head was always in the clouds was that she was quite a dreamer. Betsy wanted to be a writer!

They had spent two hours laughing, learning, and making the best-baked goods ever.

"Thank you," Sandy said to both girls, "you both taught me a lot".

"And me too", Betsy said gently, "how... how you decided to take your chances and tell your mother about the science fair... it has been news all around. I finally found the nerve to inform my mother I wanted to be a writer".

Sandy gasped

"What did she say?" Lily asked gently.

And Betsy nodded an excited yes.

*****

Sandy got permission to travel to the science fair. And oh! What a science fair it was!

*****

Aren't we all alike? More alike than we expect. We all have dreams, and that we have fears that substitute our way to achieve them. But we all got to keep determined and calculate our friends' support to get where we would like to travel.

Take a relaxing breath as you shut your eyes to sleep, ignore all distractions and let your mind focus, make your own story where you overcome your present difficulties and have your dreams come true because you're not alone.

Trip into Starlight

The night sky holds many wonders and mysteries.

For ages, we had gazed up at the stars and searched for answers to our most profound questions. Stars were utilized as maps to aid us, and He recounted many stories while they waved over us in the night.

As you delve into your long journey into your dreams and unconscious, you'll end up being taken to distant shores far away from your life on Earth and find yourself amidst several glorious visions.

Turn from the Earth around you and prepare for a trip from our world to the beyond cosmic lights.

Get yourself into the most comfortable position.

Lean into that position and scan your whole body for any tension, aches, and pains, anything you would possibly be holding onto physically.

Find those spaces and consciously release them.

Let it all accompany your breath.

Relaxation begins together with your breath, and throughout this meditation bedtime story, keeping a gentle breath will help you relax your body, mind, and heart.

You can begin with your breath by simply drawing it into your nostrils and exhaling it out of your nostrils or mouth. Inhale slowly, exhale slowly. Inhale exhale.

Your sense of calm, your serenity, your peace of mind lives in your breath.

Allow it to continue as you allow your body to completely release all of the strain you're still carrying from your day, your week, even the past several months.

Feel it vacate your body and let all of your muscles address jam or jelly.

If your muscles feel hard, soften them.

If your muscles feel tight, loosen them.

Use your breath to seek out this physical sensation.

Your body is now more elongated, your energy is smoother, your muscles are letting go of all of your current stress, and you're now a bit more relaxed than you were before.

All of your breathing throughout these moments has taken you farther into your peacefulness and quietness.

All of your inhales and exhales have loosened your grip on the day.

Now that you have relaxed, you'll begin to travel on your more significant journey into relief and healing.

Your journey begins once you exit your house.

In your mind, see yourself walking outside of your house and into the night.

You are safe and warm, and you're now standing outside of your house under the starry night sky.

The stars are bright.

There are not any lights around you.

It is black outside, apart from the starlight.

You feel enveloped by starlight as you search and see it stretching from one horizon to the other side.

The stars are endless, and there isn't a cloud in the sky.

It is clear, and you'll see all of the stars in your hemisphere.

Continuing your breath, you welcome the starlight into you as you inhale, inhaling the sensation of connection to the most transcendent unknown, the distant mysteries of the far-off galaxies beyond.

This starlight fills your whole body with each breath and invites you to take a visit to a far-off distant place, somewhere deep in the cosmos.

There is nothing to fear, for you're here to journey.

You won't harm your human body by going this far away.

You can see your journey through the vastness of your inner mind.

There are places you'll attend that you will never journey together with your human body, but tonight, you'll fly.

Tonight you're free to float away and ascend into the very best reaches of starlight.

You feel your body become weightless as you start to take off of the surface of the world.

You are not afraid to fly.

It is as if you've always known how to fly and float in this way.

It feels natural and good.

You let your body lift from this place you were standing, and as you get higher off the bottom, you are feeling yourself being pulled higher and better up into the night of stars.

When you look down, you know you won't fall.

You are in control of your flight as if you'd always done it

It is easy to do, and you're relaxed as you're taking off.

When you look down, you watch the world begin to diminish.

The farther you go up to the stars, the smaller the buildings become, the cars, the trains, the highways, the rivers, mountains, and streams all are getting smaller and farther away, more distant.

You're floating up in the starry night where you're all but you, and every star's light twinkles at you.

Earth is way away when you look behind you, and you're closer to the moon now.

The moon is welcoming and bright.

It feels small compared to the world you only came from.

It is large enough for you to take a seat upon.

You land on the surface of the moon, and you sit down, looking back at the world.

You feel as if you can see everything more clearly now.

You are distant from your problems, your cares and worries, and you'll see your life from the surface; you can feel how different it is to look at yourself and your life from this angle.

Here on the moon, you feel open and happy that you can reminisce about the world in this way and reflect.

You can contemplate here and find answers to unravel your problems and challenges.

You can see clearly from here because you're not right in it—you are closer to yourself at this moment.

You are closer to your higher purpose once you come to the present place of stillness deep in.

From here on the moon, you feel the brightness of the sun reflecting off the surface.

The silvery moonlight looks like it's wrapping itself around you, like an ethereal blanket of security and luxury.

The luminosity is recharging your batteries and helping you to feel rejuvenated and refreshed, like bathing in light. Your breath comes in, and you'll breathe easily here.

You are of the cosmos; then you'll survive in this place.

You can keep it up and go deeper into the calming serenity of Universal light.

You travel where no one on Earth can, and along with your thoughts, your subconscious, and your intuition guide you, you travel there.

You are getting to prepare to go away from the moon and travel even farther beyond.

As you get up on the surface, you feel your body bend at the knees then push you off the surface.

You begin to float out, far away from the moon, being pulled forward into the starry night, beyond Earth, beyond the moon, beyond time.

You can feel yourself getting farther and farther away, and you are feeling serene, safe, and on top of things.

You are the captain of this interstellar flight.

You are safe, and your body is capable of taking this trip.

You are here to seek out your cosmic truth.

You are here to line yourself free.

You can see your entire reality so clearly from all the answers here, far away into the starry night.

You are here to be, to exist, to enjoy the liberty that exists here.

You are burdened by nothing.

You have no obligations here.

You have only your inner power, your truth, your release from all of your current life problems and challenges. You're safe to omit all your cares, worries in the vastness of the cosmos, in the deep of space.

You are liberal to realize your most profound truth in this place in space.

You are hospitable to all things, and it feels safe and calm.

This is cool, centred.

The starlight is holding you closely, protecting you on your journey into the distant realms of space.

You are entering an area that's colourful and large.

A nebula is making ahead of your eyes, sort of a cosmic waterfall of blue and gold dotted with red and green starlight.

This starry cloud of dust opens to wish flower petals blooming on a rose.

You are invited to return closer to that and let yourself fall flat it, sort of a tunnel into another reality.

Getting closer and closer to the present massive, smoky rainbow, you start to feel pulled into it softly.

It is gentle and calm, and you're not in a hurry out here in the great beyond.

The nebula surrounds you softly, gently.

It begins to show into a tunnel that your body can float through.

You are unsure where the tunnel will lead, but you're calm and relaxed.

You don't get to know.

You are filled with the facility of the cosmos, and you're asleep in your mind and your body.

You allow your body to only glide through the nebula tunnel, feeling hospitable whatever lies beyond.

You are transported through the tunnel until you feel your body sitting on a sandy shore. You take a glance around at this space, a broad, vast landscape on another planet, somewhere in a distant galaxy.

You can feel the softness of the sand.

It is different from Earth's sand, softer, more delicate, blue-green in places, and yellow and red splotches in others.

The air is fresh here.

You can breathe easily.

You feel relaxed and calm, curiously taking in the place you have found through the tunnel.

You can feel the air is warm but not too hot.

You can feel a soft breeze that brings you into contact with a gorgeous scent in the air.

There are strange and exotic flowers and plants that look foreign, alien to you.

You are drawn to their unique qualities and colours, like nothing you have ever seen on Earth before.

Sitting here in this place, you're ready to feel the calmness of your mind, body, and heart.

You are in total peace and centeredness.

You are distant and in a place where you're safe to rest and relax.

The landscape you have found is reassuring and pleasant, and as you lie back on the softest sand, you search into the starry night sky.

You can see the galaxy far, distant that you travelled from, and you recognize that you are going to be resting there in your home when it's time to travel back.

You can leave the soft sand of this other world and start your return journey home.

You get up and take a deep breath in, pulling altogether of the beautiful serenity of this far-off distant shore.

The nebula gas returns and pulls you in, as if it never left you, as if it had always been there, expecting you to return home.

You can transcend space and time another time and travel back through the tunnel.

You find your way through the nebula tunnel with ease and beauty, moving slowly, gently.

You are getting closer and closer to space where you entered the tunnel, and as you start it, you discover yourself back in the vastness of space, covered in starlight.

You are pulled from the nebula, floating back through the cosmos the way that you came, retracing your steps through the ethereal realms of the stars.

Each breath you're taking in and exhale will push you forward to your destination.

Each inhales you the vital force you would like to propel yourself back home.

Each exhale gets you closer to your healing and relief, letting it all go and leaving it to answer here in space.

You are much closer to home now because you'll see the moon again.

You are narrowing in on the moon, and you opt to take an opportunity here before making the ultimate trip home to your house.

You float toward the surface of the moon and gracefully land, finding a cosy spot to take a seat and absorb the luminosity of the moon's surface.

You have all of the time in the Universe to only sit here and relax for a flash.

Sitting here, watching the world from the moon, you recognize your home.

From a distance, you'll relate to everything and everybody.

You can feel the earnest efforts of all people to steer a real-life and look for a more profound truth.

Looking out upon the world from this place, you remind yourself that even the most critical problems you face are little compared to the energy of all life in the Universe.

Here you'll feel refreshed, relaxed, the calm of mind and body.

You are everything and everybody, everywhere, right in this moment of reflection, all the answers here on the moon, surrounded by stars.

As you ponder the importance of your life and the lifetime of all others down there on Earth, let your breath still be slow and steady, filling you with gratitude and acceptance, letting in forgiveness and trust, patience and compassion.

When you can return, you'll float back to the world and enter your most profound comfort and rest.

You get up on the moon's surface and prepare to launch.

You push yourself off of the surface and glide slowly and peacefully toward the world.

You are following the same path you took to get up to the stars.

It will take you right back to your house, where you stood outside and searched at the starlight.

You are getting closer and closer to the Earth's surface, and the moon is becoming a distant friend again.

You can feel yourself being pulled in the right direction.

You are not in a hurry.

You are not gaining speed.

You are gently floating, flying home slowly, delicately, peacefully.

The mountains and trees, the rivers and streams are starting to become more prominent, closer, as you slowly descend back to the surface of your home planet.

You are closer now, and every one of the buildings and cars, buses, and other people are coming closer and clearer into view. Your body is slow and steady, sort of a hot air balloon, floating quietly and calmly to the bottom.

As you come closer to home, you're able to land.

You touch the surface of the world together with your toe, followed by your foot, then your other foot lands, and you're now two feet back on the bottom, back on Earth.

You turn your head to seem copy at the starry night sky.

You are home again, which was also your home for a time.

You release all of your worries and cares up there, and you're now able to walk back inside your house and end up able to fall sound asleep.

You go inside, close the door, walk to your room where you're lying down, and go deeper and deeper and deeper into sleep.

Kylie's Return to the Forest

The forest shadows swayed because as Sun continued her lazy descent.

Kylie loved it when everything was transitioning into the nighttime proceedings while the excitement of the late afternoon activities had not yet subsided.

She walked barefoot in the grass, alongside the roots, and over fallen logs, which she used as mossy bridges to cross a stream. Since she was a little girl, Kylie had come here, the advantage of having your backyard right next to the forest.

Oh, of course, when she was younger, her parents used to worry, but she was older now; she knew how to look out for herself.

Besides, the forest was her friend. Her parents never understood that part.

A golden light shone down into the clearing. Green dust glittered in the rays that splayed through the leaves. Flowers bloomed in the clearing, blues, yellows, and reds in many hundreds, and an old stump stood in the middle of the clearing.

She didn't know what had happened to the tree, but the old stump wasn't dead.

Kylie had known that since she was a child.

When she first came here and sat on the stump, she could feel it living beneath her, telling her the stories of long extended life in this place before ever there was a person's voice questioning whether the trees did make sounds once they fell!

As it clothed, the old stump had quite a lot to tell quite a while after he had fallen!

Colourful birds sang incessantly in the branches. A number of them stopped to seem at her, to chirp a greeting, and Kylie waved.

A light breeze tugged at her hair and her clothes.

She smiled and inhaled deeply. The air was so fresh in the clearing, in the forest.

She stooped and smelled some flowers. Learning a fallen red bloom, she set it in her hair and continued along the small meadow until she came to the stump.

Sitting together with her legs dangling over the stump (it had seemed so high ten years ago), Kylie sat back on her hands and searched.

One by one, tiny pinpoints of white appeared in a deepening blue canvas above.

A lone hare bounded into the clearing. It stopped and stood up, watching her, then it happily leapt away. Then a fox appeared, going the other direction, but the fox stopped to speak to her.

"Good evening," said the fox.

"Good evening," said Kylie, and she smiled, and the fox smiled.

"Where would you be going tonight?" asked the fox.

"Oh, I don't know! I assumed maybe I might just see what the forest was dreaming of tonight?"

The fox sat and lifted her nose, sniffing the air as if expecting something. "There may be a lovely feeling in the wind tonight. I desire to share. Would you wish to dream with me tonight?"

Kylie's eyes lit up. "Yes, I would! I've always wondered what foxes dreamed."

The fox laughed. "Then place your hand on my head and that I will show you."

Kylie hopped down from the stump and approached the fox.

She wondered if she should be afraid, given the fox's reputation as a trickster, but something in the air told her to go along with it.

A fantastic, comfortable night was coming, and she wanted to dream what the fox dreamed.

She placed her hand on the fox's head, her fingers threading through warm fur, and the fox laughed. "Heed no nightly noises, for tonight we dream together!"

Then Kylie leapt away in the body of the fox, and the forest came to life.

A shimmering green light appeared to emanate from the trees themselves, pulsing softly as if in tune with the land heartbeat itself.

Kylie, the fox, saw motes of glowing green: fireflies, they were, but bigger and brighter than any she had ever seen. Their light created a bit of music, and everyone things danced in tune with the music.

Flowers swayed on their stalks. The branches above waved back and forth, and the leaves fluttered, turning colours like butterfly wings then flying away.

The fox felt the music of the forest so keenly.

Perhaps that's why she was so amused: to her, every moment was a waking dream, and now Kylie needs to feel a part of that.

She felt sort of a part of the forest itself, of the endless green and growing things.

Along the paths, she darted, swifter than the hares that fled her coming, nimbler than the squirrels that skittered up the trees.

As she ran, she grew to understand the forest because the fox knew it: paws on the world, wind in the fur, the taste of freedom upon her tongue.

The night they veiled the forest in deepest blue. The lights danced in the trees and guided her way.

There were dangers, to make sure, the night spirits and the ancient ones that walked the deep forest, but they might not catch her.

She was the fox, too quick and too sly for anyone to catch her.

Because she knew the tune for all of them, it gave her a unique guidance strategy as she bounded through the woods.

Fox had the quickest feet and the fastest wits.

She had never been caught yet in many long, long years, and she wasn't getting to be now.

Kylie felt confidence and a way of utter peace.

She was united with the land itself, with the dream, with both waking and sleeping worlds, flesh and blood, root and sap, reality and fantasy.

She was a part of this great music, familiar on the main primal level, directly the foremost ancient and always a new scent, sound, taste, and feel. She knew the sheer joy of darting from bush to bush, path to path, racing into an entire night of potential.

Howls went up into the night because the wolves were closed, but the pack came not as enemies.

She ran among them for a time, fellow travellers in the forest night-dream.

The only sounds were of panting breaths and paws thumping on the world in time with the land's pulse for that span.

They were all one, a glimpse of the sheer exultant joy of life in its most early incarnation. Blood thundered. Voices howled.

The night was alive around them; spirits capered in the wind and half-hidden in the shadowy eaves.

Some looked on with laughter at the passing four-legs, some looked on with envy, but none could match their sense of pure freedom.

The moment passed, and the fox went her way amid howls of kinship from the wolves, for she had far to travel yet before the Sun rose and dispelled the magic of the night.

The deep forest was an area of the foremost ancient and primal dreams.

Here stood trees that had outlasted ages of the planet, groves that had way back disappeared in the waking world but remained hale and bountiful here.

They were sustained by and embodied the very dreams of the land itself, a time of rampant growth and viridian tenacity.

Their voices were deep and hollow when they sang, ringing far out over the land, heard by every leaf and stem. Needles danced upon the forest floor at its vibration, and leaves upon the branches fluttered happily.

Shadows were deep beneath the tall trees, but they hid neither malice nor dangers.

The forest's deepest heart was an area of pure growth, where the most important of the trees would count its rings more significant than the number of leaves in the forest.

Each of the mighty trees bore a whole world upon its branches. As a fruit, these visions hung a globe, storm, and an ocean in a single drop.

If one dropped, it burst into life and filled all the dreams of the forest.

From root to treetop, the good trunks emanated this music of creation, bastions of a time when the planet was young and its harmonies still coming together.

Like the fox, she bounded happily through these forest depths, privy as few sleepers were to the powerful sounds of the most ancient of living things.

The land itself spoke through these guardians, and everyone who would know the reality of the dreaming earth could listen.

Few experiences were more transformative, and Kylie may have lingered for a lifetime or several to concentrate.

"It is amazing," said Fox. "You are fortunate. Not many can hear this music conducted from the guts of the forest. It's the facility to shape the planet itself."

"I know," said Kylie, her voice hazy as if caught in the spell of sleep. "It's old but ageless, sort of a new pebble abruption of a mountain. Alternatively, a drop from the waterfall, it's a part of something impossibly old, but also touches you wish it had been fresh."

Fox laughed. "You speak well, friend. This is often the song that courses through the lifeblood of the planet. What you feel when your feet touch the nice and cozy grass in the summertime, otherwise you smell the air after a rain; otherwise, you feel the breeze that blows warm through the forest. This place is the very embodiment of that feeling. Life is at its strongest here, and its dreams are the most potent."

Kylie could have spent forever absorbing that potency, but she had such a lot more she wanted to ascertain.

Together with Fox, they hurtled roots and fallen branches and leapt across shallow ravines.

They passed clearings where the daylight never left, even at the deepest of night.

Those were places where the planet had been awake for so long that wakefulness and dreaming were equal things.

Tinged with the primal essence of living history, the sunlit clearings warmed Fox's fur, but she hurried through them. "There are other places I would like to point out to you yet before we see the Sun again!"

The paths that led through the forest would have left most travellers hopelessly lost, wandering in the great emerald great thing about the forest until they awakened.

The fox was sly, and she knew the paths better than anyone.

She couldn't easily get lost, even in the depths of the forest.

Over hills and across ravines upon moss-covered fallen logs, she darted, swift and sure.

Her nose lifted into the air sometimes to snuff out the trail, or her ears flicked as she stopped to concentrate, but she always found her way.

She had run the forest for several long years, and she would still do so for several more to return.

At last, the cover thinned again, and she came to more minor wild parts of the woods.

She came to a stream bubbling and gushing along a well-worn path.

The fox turned her course, running alongside it for several miles.

The stream spoke to her because it rushed and burbled along its path, envious of her ability to settle on her path, carrying many voices from distant lands.

"Hello!" said the fox to the stream. "Are you cold and swift tonight?"

"I am cold and swift," said stream, "but I carry many dreams! Maybe one will warm you?"

There was an airing into the edible water and being taken away as part of its continuous stream of dreams and voices.

"Not tonight!" laughed Fox, and she jumped clear over the stream.

Its voice faded behind her as she saw the deeper forest and raced up an excellent grassy hill.

Capitol Hill's top reached just above the tree line so that it appeared to be a green head crowned in trees.

Fox saw a sea of deep green all-round her, faintly illuminated by silver starlight above and green earthlight beneath. "This! This is often the best view in the forest. But this happens only in the deepest hours, just before the Sun returns." Then Kylie was herself again, beside the fox, and looking out upon a similar fantastic view.

There was one broad stump on the highest of Capitol Hill, and she sat upon it, dangling her legs, breathlessly admiring the incredible view.

Like every dream, the forest had been woven into a perfect tapestry.

"So, does one regret running with me?" asked Fox.

Nevertheless, she already knew the solution that never came because Kylie was sound asleep, curled on the stump, and sleeping more soundly than she had in a few years.

Fox smiled, for she had long to travel yet, but Kylie's journey ended here.

She had more to pass through, more dreams to seek out, but tonight, Kylie slept because the forest itself did.

Fox darted into the shadow of the woods.

Fireflies danced in the air Kylie, who dreamed of running sort of a fox through the magical forest.

* * *

"Did you actually get to sleep in the forest with the foxes and the trees and the fireflies, Mommy?"

Jenny smiled. "Yes, dear. Now, tonight you'll get to do the same thing."

Nevertheless, the small girl was already asleep, with a smile on her face.

Jenny tucked the blankets in around her and shut off the lights, pausing to smile.

Alone in the Space

Before we start this journey into the deepest realms of our subconscious, allow us to take a moment to physically, mentally, and spiritually acclimate ourselves into being with the awareness of our inner sanctum, our internal workings. We'll start by going to an area of comfort, ideally a bed or a comfortable recliner, and we will relax our bodies to the furthest extent possible.

Now, close your eyes, laying on your back, with your arms relaxed at your sides and your legs rested downwards. Take one deep breath in, through your nostrils, counting slowly to four, and one deep breath out, through your nostrils again, counting slowly to four. Inhale the breath of the Spirit and exhale the strain of the day.

Now's the time to rest! Become conscious of nothing but the air flowing through your nostrils; envision a gently flowing stream, smooth inhalations and exhalations, your body become weightier and more relaxed with each passing cycle of breath. Allow your thoughts to become completely still as you concentrate on your core, your coeliac plexus. Allow your ideas to flow outwards past your vision until they escape your being while only holding and retaining the pure awareness of Spirit, the holy serenity of the mind and body. Inhale, one, two, three, four, then exhale, one, two, three, four, each breath becoming slower.

One... two... three... four... One... two... three... four... One... two... three... four... One... two... three... four... One... two... three... four... One... two... three... four...

Continue this pattern of breath, expanding, and sink deeper into yourself, becoming a voyeur of your own still, relaxed body, lost in time. Lost yourself in this experience as you travel further into the trance and prepare yourself for the path you are about to take. Draw further away from your still, lying body and into the realm of imagination, where images grow, the land of dreams that you are close to becoming one with. Erase your mind of all that's in it currently, and prepare the landscape for a new and fresh experience in the farther reaches of reality.

One... two... three... four... inhale... One... two... three... four... exhale... One... two... three... four... inhale... One...

two... three... four... exhale...

Now, with your mind, body, and Spirit rested, entranced, and fertile, let us start.

The mountains stretch forever, in every direction. Civilization exists in another place and a few other times.

Here, now, it's only you.

You're flowing downstream, endlessly, on a raft of your design, with blankets, and zip to occupy your thoughts or your feelings besides your surroundings, and the sensation itself, of floating, forever, lackadaisically, relaxed, at a snail's pace, down this stream, this vein flowing through the guts of the world, all the blood of life passing through, effortlessly, slowly, from the courage and back again.

You do not remember when or where you started, and you have no idea when or where it'll end, just that it'll be a very while and a very, very long way away. The repetition of the scenery hypnotizes you, yet, somehow, each new area is so pleasantly new in some subliminal way, you are feeling endlessly entertained, like some enchanted treadmill of the soul, you'll watch these repeating trees, huddled together, endlessly, for the remainder of your life. You'd be perfectly content, each new grouping of trees, each new formation of rock you pass, each shore, so unique in its way, feeding your soul in a sustainable cycle. You become familiar with these repeated stimuli, and it creates new homeostasis in your mental being of perfect satisfaction.

The breeze is steady, soft kisses on your exposed skin and the flow of the river are endless, yet wild, in a pleasant, relaxing way. There are swoops and sways, and every stretch of the river is entirely different from the last, yet so familiar, then endless, then assuring in its repeated, steady flow downwards.

Sometimes the river is wilder, pushing you up and down like little hills, little waves knocking around your raft, surfing along with them, wondering if you may be flung off, yet you never are, so you become more and more relaxed, increasing your comfort level.

Then, sometimes, the river is more calm and peaceful, almost as if it's bringing your raft to a standstill. But these sections are as enjoyable and vital as they enable us to take the vast countryside, the trees, the bushes, even the heavens, and your inner landscapes, and your life and body, blood and soul, to an ideal size.

In one of these long, peaceful passages, you notice a family of deer, and, taking advantage of the calm river before them, they cross right ahead of your raft. You say hello to them, and they check you out, and it humbles you to realize that they are comfortable together with your presence; it causes you to be delighted.

You're feeling considerable as if you are totally at one with nature. You feel as if you are a part of this river, sort of a branch, having fallen off a tree an extended way back, being taken down the river wherever it's going to go, being digested by the world somewhere along the way, taken in, absorbed, and given back in some new make, somewhere copy the road, of space, and time.

The perpetual cycle of things is highly apparent to you here on this trip. This river itself is relatively the river of your time. Down and down, it keeps going, never-ending, an endless forest surrounding it, endless places for it to travel. While it goes, it carves a path, and the way becomes new things, and life is given along the trail, by the waters, and life is taken down the course, by the waters, and brought elsewhere. Where it goes, nobody knows.

Endlessly down the river, down, down, and down, into the ocean, then, somehow, back again, back to the peak of the mountain only to eventually succumb to the river, relaxed, letting the river take it down, sleeping, down around to rock bottom.

So is life, so is the nature of all things. Here, where you're, now, you're on a journey back to the rock bottom, back to the well. On this journey, it's your job only to relax. All the work is behind you. Now the river is doing all the work that's to be finished you, by the water's flowing, by time itself. By the top, you'll be at rock bottom, and you'll be placed sweetly back to the ocean if there even is an end, which, to you now, is unknowable. As you're not consciously conscious of the start, you're also not consciously aware of the top, only the character of all things. Therefore, you should know that eventually, somewhere along the road, everything must end and return to wherever it came from. It's difficult for you in your state to focus on the after that and the eternal downstream.

Day turns into night, repeatedly, and the noises from the forest take suit. The sunshine green fauna of the day turns into a dark web of mystery in the dark.

You see glowing eyes peering from the trees, and here low growls, and footsteps, wild beasts stalking in the night, as you float endlessly past. Within their natural habitat, the rubbish and gobbling were happening in the eternal forest, besides you, as you travel through, a passenger through and out the stream.

Days travel by, and you stare fixedly, allowing the passing forest to warp into some hypnotizing blur.

The noises of the wild encounter you, as if the embodiment of the forest is a few spirits, besides you in the raft, whispering playfully to you, fantastic, grand nothings. You laugh, tease a joke being told to you by the good Spirit, and you yawn. Your eyelids become heavy as another transition into the dark mystery of the night begins. Aside from you, as you journey through life, down the stream, relaxed, on your back, body rested, and cosy, and still, feeling for eternity the soft rocking of the raft on the infinite waters, the stream of consciousness flowing forever down the mountain. You close your eyes, listen to the tears of the forest and the rustle of the wind in the blades, make your mind more comfortable in a better condition, distant from yourself, down, into dreams.

Blue Ocean

Some days seem as if they will never be over. Days where it looks like your entire life will end, as every activity is done, takes a toll on you, from your annoying boss to some annoying customers.

This has been my daily routine. My nights are not any different. My heart burns from the excessive caffeine I need to keep me working. Life isn't as easy as I assumed it might be. I had my entire life mapped out with set goals and achievements to accumulate. I always strive for the best, but the best never comes easy.

Gone are the times where you had someone do all the housework, prepare your breakfast, and you can wake up like a king or queen. Being an adult isn't as easy as I assumed. Now I yearn for the times by the ocean, with a cool breeze and the singing waves, the flip flop sound as dolphins delve from one point to another, just that sanity, where my head can filter out from these emotional drama and life affairs.

These thoughts ran through my head as I walk around the hospital lobby. My youngest son has been diagnosed with lung cancer; we were told he had a couple of months to survive.

A few minutes later, I would be in Kanye's ward. His bed was by the window, where he has a view where he can lookout. He spends a large part of his day doing that. Today was no different as I met him in his wheelchair beside his window; his nurse attended him.

Kanye may be weak for nature's gentle touch; he's either gazing out of his window or reading one of his books. They were always books about nature. Kanye would always ask, Mama, why don't we have a house by the ocean? Have you ever seen a dolphin before? Why is the wind by the sea cooler than the wind we've got here? Do oceans end? Can they ever dry up?

He would always say, "I want to be just like the ocean; when am I able to see one?"

Lost in my thoughts, I heard him call "mummy." "Your eyes are heavy," he said.

Can I be your Blue Ocean?

I looked deep into his blue eyes. It reminds me of a rhyme from a page in his book. I picked him up and lay him on his bed, and he sat up straight; he rested his back on the soft and delicate pillow, picked up his book, and looked for that page. He reads;

I hear you call from upon the waters; my heart skips as your voice roars like the waves of the ocean. I see your eyes, so blue. My heavy heart wishes for you to remain calm.

My feet are wobbling, and my body is shaking. My nights are scary; my eyes are teary and dreary. I want your touch to help calm my storm.

But when my heart rises just like the ocean, who will calm this storm?

The breeze blows; I can hear the peace. So I'm calm as I rest in its embrace.

As he reads, I lay my head beside him as I pictured every word he says. I could imagine us holding hands as Kanye runs toward the ocean just a few feet away; he laughs hard as he steps into the shore. The waves come and splash him. For once, I saw my Kanye in a different way, not a dying child, but one filled with life. Somehow I find peace. Indeed, you're my ocean.

Taking Flight in Dreamland

Nearly all of us have had a dream that we are flying.

Sometimes you have wings.

Sometimes you're just gliding through the air like some superhero.

Dreaming is symbolic of freedom and allows us to let go of our fears.

Flying has been described in the legends of old myths and folktales describing a flying person as having special powers.

Your dreams will always lead you to a sort of self-discovery in which you're taking control of your journey, your destiny. You're the captain, and you recognize precisely where to fly, how high, and when to land.

Planting your feet on the land all day is often complex, especially if you have a challenging or difficult situation or people in your life or if you have a tough time processing your feelings and emotions.

Guided meditations and artistic visualization are an enormous part of what makes enlightened people find their way to wholeness.

Your inner journey is as valuable, meaningful, and essential as your inner one.

When you follow your journey forward and trust yourself to fly in the right direction for yourself, then the stresses of life naturally fall away, and you'll find peace, harmony, and balance together with your whole life. So take a flash to attach with this positive notion.

Find your temperature, and let yourself fall under freely.

You are here to enjoy your life journey, not stress out about it all of the time.

You are here to possess a purpose that's meaningful to you, not worry about whether or not you're doing an honest enough job or if you're successful enough.

You have always been and always are enough, and once you acknowledge that truth, that's once you can fly.

Find your most comfortable position.

Find the parts of your body that feel restless or tense and shake them out.

Shake out any part of your body that has felt motionless for much too long.

Shake off any annoyance about another person today or any challenging experiences. Shake off all of the drama that finds you once you try to seek out your peace of mind.

Inhale deeply and breathe; gain control over your breath.

Exhale slowly and appreciate the way it feels to release something physically from your body.

Inhale slowly again, rejoicing in the fresh air that fills you up.

Exhale slowly and feel gratitude that you have come to the present place of self-healing, to bond together with your creative inspiration and thoughts, to become even more closely connected to your inner self, free from drama, free from critique. No one is judging you.

Your breath has helped your body feel more relaxed.

You are sinking more deeply into your comfort and relaxation.

You are finding it easier to breathe naturally and smoothly.

You feel content to be present here, taking excellent care of yourself, giving yourself all of the love, attention, and devotion you need immediately.

There are not any rules on your inner journey.

All you have to do is appreciate your creative ability to ascertain more clearly from your inner world.

Sometimes, all you would like is to travel in to seek out your answers and flee, resolving all of your problems, issues, and challenges from your internal self.

You are fully relaxed as you still breathe, and let yourself take comfort in your power and light from within.

You may desire you have already done this before, and that's okay.

You don't need to believe any of it—you need to let yourself follow along, hear the guided story, and enjoy the pleasure of flying.

You can see yourself now.

You are watching your reflection in a mirror or a window.

You can see your face, your features, and your outfit.

How would you wish to feel right now?

Do you feel the way you look in your reflection in your mind?

Do you look the way that you hope to feel?

As you looked at your inner reflection, show yourself how you would like to seem to yourself.

Give yourself the costume or design or outfit that most accurately fits how you would like to feel tonight.

You can change your hairstyle.

You can wear something you'd typically never prefer to place on publicly.

Take a couple of moments as you breathe to understand the planet you recognize in your mind.

You can be all of yourself here.

Allow yourself to seem the way you'd wish to feel immediately.

You are getting to desire this for the remainder of your guided meditation.

It is your world, and you'll look and dress; however you see fit.

You can change your outfit anytime you would like to.

You can become whatever you are at heart inside.

You might become an animal or a tree.

You might become a warrior or a princess.

You might become something that this world has never known before.

Enjoy the work of dressing yourself to fly.

When you are ready, inhale deeply, hold your breath for a count of three, and steadily release the breath from your body.

You are climbing up a staircase now.

It is made from stone, and it's carved as a spiral, going higher and better.

It looks just like the stairs in an ancient castle.

The castle may be a part of your subconscious.

It is an area you'll come to any time you would like to decorate yourself the way you would like to or hope to feel inside and out.

The stairs are taking you up to the highest of the castle.

When you get to the rooftop, you're ready to walk out onto it.

The castle overlooks an excellent and vast kingdom.

It is familiar to you.

You have travelled here before.

As you look out over the land, you'll think about other places you've already been: in a meadow, in a forest, by the ocean on a ship, in the clouds, by a river, in a garden of wonders.

This place holds the critical truth of you and your inner journey.

The landscape is wholly yours; you'll be anything here, and you can do anything you would like to assist yourself find your truth and purpose.

It is where you'll return as you go after deeper meaning in your life, as you seek to understand who you are, at heart inside.

Standing on the castle roof, taking in the inner world of your mind, you're now ready to take a new journey.

From here in your kingdom, you'll fly anywhere.

You are dressed to be how you would like to feel, you have all of your inner power and life force to guide you, and you'll fly over everything and everybody to get to your space of balance, harmony, and equality with the life you would like to be living.

The flight will take you far, and the point of your journey now's to let your intuition guide you.

Your inner wisdom can help you find what you would like to ascertain immediately to help you relax and find peace of mind and inner calm.

You can let yourself find the right path once you trust that you already know the answers.

You already skills to unravel all of your problems, and you'll find it alright here in this inner kingdom of your body, mind, heart, and soul.

To take flight, all you have to do is face the planet you have created in your thoughts and mind.

Take a flash to breathe and relax into this visual journey.

Take a flash to attach with your breath again and let yourself feel that moment before you're taking flight. Stepping closer to the roof's edge, imagine you're outstretching your arms like their wings, stretching far bent on either side of you.

Underneath, you're just castle grounds, or is it a waterfall that leads through an excellent misty fog that goes to a different place in your kingdom?

When you look down, you see not the grounds of a castle but a portal into another place, and you'll fly there just by leaping off the rooftop and finding your flight.

The waterfall drops off into another place you can't see.

It is where you'll begin to show yourself the way to journey in your mind.

You can imagine anything you would like, anything in the least.

You can see beyond the truth of Earth and its appearance in your inner universe with creativity and imagination.

You can picture a rainbow bridge to fly over, which will lead you to a different part of your kingdom.

You can picture a flying Pegasus who will transport you wherever you would like to travel.

Here, in your kingdom, there are not any rules.

You are the one who decides how your world will look and the way you'll find your way forward.

So, now, here in this place, prepare to take a flight.

Your arms are spread.

Your outfit is simply right.

You are relaxed, calm, and liberal to be anything you would like.

Push off and fly go wherever your intuition is guiding you.

You will not fall.

You will not be hurt.

You have the power to fly in this place, and you're liberal to make your way through this world together with your secret wing-span.

As you're taking flight and your world exposes to you more, what does one find? What are you able to see?

Are there others here?

Are there new lands yet to be explored — more hidden caves and majestic gardens or more cosy cottages deep in the woods, or ships to be sailed over your private ocean?

Do any animal guides join you?

Enjoy flying over your inner kingdom, and let it keep unfolding for you.

Breathe steadily.

You can land anywhere you would like and begin anywhere you would like.

You are flying to get a much bigger picture; greater scope and zip are just too big or too small here.

It is everything you ask it to be.

[Give much time for creative visualization and meditation here]

Your world is an awakening place.

It helps you discover your creative life force, your more profound truth, your purpose.

This world within your mind may be a sacred landscape, a dimension of your thoughts and feelings, to be explored as a great adventurer seeking hidden treasure in every cave, forest, and hideaway.

Bring your focus back to your breath.

Let yourself continue exploring in ways you'll not have before.

Let yourself delve more deeply into these ascended places.

Who does one meet along the way?

Have you met another spirit guide or ascended master who teaches you a lesson of healing and spiritual wisdom?

Do you have any specific places that you feel more drawn to in this unique universe?

Wherever you're in your flight, give yourself a flash to ascertain if you'll find your castle again from now of view.

Can you tell where you're on the map of your mind?

Are there secret tunnels and portals which will lead you right back to your castle?

Begin to seek out your way back to the castle now, breathing steadily and slowly along the way.

You can see it, and it feels far, but you have the power to fly.

It won't take long to get there.

You are feeling more peaceful now and prepared to fall sound asleep.

Your journey through the dominion has shown you much and given you much to understand.

You will find your sense of relaxation and restfulness more fully now.

You will feel able to align together with your dreaming mind and drift further and further into sleep.

The castle is drawing nearer, and you are feeling yourself preparing to land.

You have a robust body and are good at landing from your flight.

It is a dance, graceful and angelic.

The castle roof welcomes you back with ease, and you are feeling powerfully connected to your higher nature.

You follow your original path back to the mirror where you initially began.

Down, down, down the stone steps of the castle, such as you are unwinding.

As you come to the mirror again, you see your eyes again, face, and body.

You see your outfit.

It may have changed, and that's okay.

Or perhaps, after flying through your inner world, you're able to accept a new form.

How does one want to decorate now, as you steel oneself against a wholesome night of gentle, peaceful rest?

What would feel best to you immediately after touching the liberty of flight?

Take a couple of moments and breaths to ascertain yourself in the castle mirror.

Now, you're ready.

You can now retire in your inner kingdom, in the castle of your dreams and imagination.

Not far from your glass may be a large bed, fit a queen or king.

It has the softest sheets and blankets, the deepest, most comfortable pillows, and it's all for you, expecting you, warm and alluring.

You beat and climb high to the massive mattress, tucking your legs under the covers, feeling silk against your skin.

You can finally rest after an extended flight and journey around your kingdom.

As you snuggle in, long, heavy velvet curtains are pulled closed around the bed, wrapping you in comfort and deep, luxurious peacefulness.

You are liberal to disappear into your dreams now.

Your work is completed.

You are here to rest all the way, deep into the planet of the unconscious.

Release your breath feel held by the magic of your castle, your kingdom, your inner world. You can fly anywhere you would like, even into your dreams.

You are floating into your dreams now, soft and serene, high in your castle, safe, wrapped in velvet and silk, dream that you simply are flying over your kingdom again peacefully, serenely, calmly sweet dreams.

Winter Dreams

Rhoda watched because the snow continued to fall and mount outside the window.

Fog lightly obscured the window.

She reached up to rub a number of it away, her fingers squeaking on the cold glass.

A steaming mug of hot cocoa warmed her hands, and she curled her fingers around the warm face. Another profile sat on the windowsill beside her.

The lights were low in the front room, apart from the fireside, which crackled with a merry fire. Shadows danced across space.

Clara lay on the ground ahead of the hearth, resting her chin in her hands, watching the shapes that formed and melted away even as quickly in flames.

Soft holiday music played on a speaker.

Clara hummed alongside it.

The snow finally began to slow. Larger flakes fell lazily upon a city blanketed in white.

The steady sound of a snow shovel scraping on the driveway kept Rhoda's thoughts occupied.

Her husband was out there, shovelling. It had been only snow, but it had been cold enough that she worried.

At last, the scraping sounds ceased, and the snowfall dwindled to just about nothing.

The front entrance opened, and a tall man with a shawl around his neck, a white-flecked wool hat, and red cheeks stepped in.

Rhoda picked up the cup of cocoa and met him at the door.

She helped him get his coat, hat, and scarf off, then handed him the mug.

"Welcome back, hon. it looks like it's finally stopped."

He took the mug and sipped slowly from it, blowing wisps of steam away.

"Oh, you usually make the best cocoa, babe. How does one do that? I can never catch on nearly as good as yours!"

He went bent the front room and sat on the ground near Clara, who also had some cocoa—though the women were maybe more marshmallows than cocoa at this point!

Rhoda retrieved her cup and joined them.

"At least it wasn't regrettable, this time. Not like last year!"

"Last year was awesome!" Clara exclaimed.

Rhoda laughed. "Oh, no, my dear. It wasn't! We were snowed under for 2 days! Don't you remember when your father broke the snow shovel? We couldn't do anything!"

"Nuh-uh, Mommy! Remember how I tunneled out of the downstairs bathroom window?"

"Don't you ever do anything like that again! That was dangerous!"

Despite herself, Rhoda smiled. The girl was undoubtedly irrepressible. Snow, rain, none of it slowed her down. However, the last winter had been pretty concerning, so Rhoda made bound to refill on firewood and candles.

Her husband stood up and went out through the back sliding door to fetch more firewood.

Rhoda had a thought. "Why don't we do a family story night, ahead of the fire? Would you wish that, sweetie?" "YES!" The girl's shriek of affirmation could have caused an avalanche!

"Okay, baby, but keep it down! Your sister is asleep. Let me go get the book."

Rhoda stood up and slipped out of the space, heading back through the front room to the steps. She had left the storybook up in Clara's room.

While she was upstairs, she stopped to see the baby; the monitor was quiet, but she just wanted to make sure.

The daughter was asleep and looked happy and peaceful.

Rhoda smiled and went back downstairs.

Clara was sitting up now, excitedly rocking back and forth while her father accumulated wood near the fireside.

She begged him to let her put in the next one, and he handed her a bit of chopped wood.

Clara zealously tossed it into the hearth, leaving her father having to adjust it quickly.

Having done that,

they both sat back, their faces aglow in the firelight.

Clara came and sat next to them, all sharing one big blanket, sitting back against the front of the couch. She set the book down on her lap.

"Okay, you two." Rhoda smiled knowingly.

"I think I even have the right story for this type of night."

She opened the book and flipped to a page showing a gorgeous snow-covered landscape.

Peaks of purest white rose into a pale blue.

The plains of snow that spread across the page glowed with cool white light, filling the front room, mingling with the golden firelight above their heads like an aurora.

In the ice, a crack had formed, looking like a "7."

"This one is going to take us to someplace that'll feel familiar ...."

A biting wind blew across the vast plains of glittering white.

Dusty snow stirred on the surface layer. Huge drifts had built up over months and formed a hilly terrain of round white hills, jagged peaks, and smoothly blanketed valleys.

Here and there, the tundra peeked through the snow, dark green mottled spots against the bluish-white scenery. Whilst the sun shone down, the snow and ice sparkled as if studded with diamonds. It had been cold but beautiful beyond measure.

Jaina stood at the peak of the small ridge and shaded her eyes.

She wrapped the headscarf around her neck and smiled.

What a view it was!

So like the snow-covered cars, driveways, and yards she had seen before she visited bed, having shovelled the driveway for the third time that day.

It was an incredible view, and she would never dream of there having to shovel and remove all the snow from this place.

Her boots crunched in the snow as she walked.

Her breath steamed in the air, curling away in wispy fingers.

The cold reddened her skin but didn't harm her; she walked among the land, as did a traveller through a dream: present but ethereal, safely experiencing another world.

She could inhale deeply and feel the ache in her lungs from the cold, dry air, and yet it didn't hurt.

Instead, it added a way of life to the setting, gave her a more incredible feeling of immersion in the blindingly bright arctic lands.

To untrained eyes, the place looked barren, but those that could see beyond the surface saw a whole world of life—tufts of green shrubs and thick carpets of lichen and moss covered much of the bottom.

While the snow was piling into and around the vegetation, something was always going on in the coldest areas; new things in the tundra evolved.

A family of white-furred hares peeked their heads up over one of the snow dunes.

They appeared to notice Jaina but didn't mind, rather chittering excitedly among themselves.

They had found some food and shared it as a family: two adult hares and two younger ones.

Their fur was so soft and fluffy; He could make it from fresh-fallen snow in itself.

Once they had finished eating as a family, all of them bounded away, soon disappearing into a burrow made into the snow berms.

They nestled down in their cosy den to enjoy the remainder of the day.

Jaina hopped along, feeling as carefree and light-footed as a hare.

It was hard not to feel the light-hearted spirit of the happy little creatures in such a bright and delightful land.

She came to a chasm, where snow looked over cliffs of a pale, luminous blue ice.

The wind whistled and howled through the chasm.

Her footstep disturbed a pile of snow, which tumbled down into the blue abyss, and she smiled. Its mysteries called to her.

She couldn't resist the temptation to take a glance.

When Jaina stepped down, her reflection in the ice fractured into thousands of different images, all grinning back at her as she drifted downward light as a snowflake.

The ice walls appeared to hold mysteries of their frozen dream-shapes and glimpses through a lens into distant worlds.

One object half-hidden in the thick ice looked like an elephant-like creature, locked in its icy dreams.

Jaina reached out and touched the ice, and suddenly she found herself transported to an ancient yet familiar land.

The giant furred beast walked because the king of the land, unchallenged in its pride and power.

Tundra opened up before it, but because the warmer months had caused a lot of ice to melt, a vast realm of green and yellow sprawled across the horizon.

Ice formed peaks and capped hills, but the land grew even amid all the ice and snow.

Hares leapt from dune to dune, becoming a part of the snow for brief moments as they vanished into the flaky puffs.

Snow owls flew over the snow, their feathers impossibly bright, like shafts of pure light radiating from their wings. Jaina watched in fascination as they flew past, their round eyes like miniature suns, shining beams before their path.

She wanted to succeed in out, but they were too fast and too high for her to succeed in, whilst the enormous.

Still, all fled her path as she walked from sunrise to sunset, then crouched to sleep the night away.

Jaina drifted far away from the frozen giant, smiling.

She had gotten to take part in his dreams and loved every second of it.

However, her own called. Jaina floated upward, rising with a sudden updraft out of the chasm, buoyed by the crisp arctic air.

She spread her arms wide and spun as she lifted, spiralling up into the daylight.

There was such a lot more to ascertain and neutralize such an area, this endlessly breathtaking land of snow and wonder.

A shrill, piping cry greeted her as she noticed a herd of thundering caribou past.

They sang as they ran together, a song of unity and hope, always excited for what lay over the next hill, just over the next horizon.

They were a family, shaggy-coated and covered in frost, but they were always there for each other.

As the herd ran, they shuddered and shifted positions, with the young in the middle of the pack.

Each raised their voice as they came to their new position. So too did their footsteps and their snorting breaths increase the more incredible music of the arctic wonderland.

For a time, Jaina ran with them, her feet gracefully skimming the highest of the snow.

She felt more vital to belong to the herd and be part of an enormous family out there in the open tundra.

Sometimes, they had only one another to believe for warmth, support, companionship, and as a part of that, Jaina felt a sense of camaraderie she had rarely experienced.

She felt more vital to be a part of the herd, all helping keep the others running lightly and happily.

Their dreams were that of the land itself: endless plains of white and green, enough food to fill every belly in the herd, and a starry sky in the dark to guide their slumber.

They welcomed the moon as much as they did the sun, and they enjoyed the bounties that the land gave freely. Theirs was a rugged existence, simple, a family together in the beautiful northern wilderness.

Jaina bade them farewell and ran on as they turned away and ran eastward.

She saw that the land soon gave way to a shelf and beyond it the frigid but alluring arctic waters.

Jaina stooped and dipped her fingers into the crystalline water, sending out a series of ripples that even rang with a high, clear note.

Simultaneously, the whole arctic sea came to life with equivalent music; each crest splashed like a ringing instrument playing a delightful tune.

Far out from the ice-locked shore, an excellent shape emerged from the water.

It gleamed like onyx, with great white spots upon its head and a belly as white as snow. Jaina cheered as more appeared.

They were orcas, one of her favourite sorts of animals, an enormous family of all of them journeying alongside the currents.

One by one, as they surfaced, each spouted, and the spouts rose like mists of the many colours, and a haunting song played because the droplets rained backtrack to the surface again.

The pod of orcas arced gracefully through the waves and the ripples they sent out, joining with those Jaina had created.

Then the whales dove and vanished again into the cold waters, and Jaina wanted quite anything to follow them did.

The sun began to sink, and she hopped out onto the ice floes, springing lightly from one to the other, hoping to get another glimpse of the orcas.

The wake of their passage left an easy trail, but Jaina couldn't seem to stay up with them. There! One breached the surface not too distant from the floes as if to point out to her they were nearby.

The waves cast by its huge body impacting sent the ice floes bobbing unsteadily, and Jaina stepped off into the cold waters. Downward she plunged in a cloud of bubbles, her bright eyes seeking a glimpse of what she loved.

She swam quickly, as if floating through the air itself, and located herself faced with the top magnificent sight she had ever seen.

Rays of faint light splayed down from the shimmering surface.

In the flowing currents deeper down, the sunshine became like clouds of luminous mist.

She dove further down, following the orcas that in the dim and refracting light seemed to be made from the night sky itself.

The light became undulating ribbons of the many colours, stretched across a vast sky that rolled like ocean waves.

Tiny pinpoints of brightest white appeared on the surface, and she realized that she swam among the orcas through an ocean of stars.

Here, because the aurora borealis filled the heavens with their mysterious glow, the borders between sea and sky had vanished completely.

The orcas were vessels congested with the stars, and so were her eyes.

They flew together into the aurora, and the sounds of their joyful, haunting songs blended with Jaina's laughter. Ripples of their harmony spread across the aurora, which danced in the night.

Jaina and the pod of orcas drifted through the atmospheric orchestra as conductors and listeners alike.

She became enveloped in the ethereal colours: green and pale blue, even red.

The sky was aflame with pure light, an area where the dreaming mind was the reality, and the song of the planet itself dispelled the waking world.

Jaina had never known such bliss as she releases all of her worries and has become one with a bit of music as old as the planet itself.

The orcas flew about her, leaping, spinning, and drifting alongside her.

To them, this was the night sky lit by the aurora as they experienced it, but Jaina was new to such a perspective. Now that she had known it, she could never sleep an equivalent way again.

Great notes formed in the aurora, carrying the sleeping night through and welcoming the approaching dawn.

Jaina and her fellow dreamers slept soundly in the sky, held aloft by the original ancient and primal songs.

Nothing could disturb their rest, as they became another part of the grandest composition.

All who searched and saw the aurora found their hopes and dreams buoyed an equivalent way, moved to float amid a cosmic chorus from which one could only know peace.

Snowcaps

I gazed at the winding trail before me.

I was completely alone on my hike.

My trip was a chance to reconnect with nature.

I needed a getaway from my lifestyle, which seemed more and more like a fishbowl.

It was free from the nagging pressures of my job and home life.

I was a toddler of nature, able to reaffirm my bond.

For the past month, I even have seen myself making this hike (in my head) nightly before I nod off.

In my mind, I even have been trekking to the very peak and searching out over the ethereal landscape.

I have felt the wind against my cheek and heard the racing river.

I have imagined warming my hands against the hearth at my camp while looking into a wild night sky filled with twinkling stars and mystery.

The mountain air was chilly and exhilarating.

I held my arms bent to my sides so that I could more fully inhale the freshness that I had been looking for goodbye. Nothing could compare to the embrace of nature.

He built our bodies to tune into the frequencies of wilderness.

The trail that I used to be trekking began a brief distance from the bottom of the mountain.

I would be finding my way to the top to line up camp.

It was an intensely scenic area in Washington State.

It sat upon the heartbeat of mother nature, a testament to the sweetness of our world.

I had brought all the required gear for climbing and camping near the peak of the mountain.

A heavy backpack caused me to hunch slightly as I walked, but I was accustomed to the load.

I would surely be thankful for my preparedness when the time came for rest.

I took a sip from my bottle and returned it to its place among my things.

My path was surrounded by woodlands, all the way to the top of the mountain.

It felt like complete isolation from the remainder of humanity.

The closest town was a quaint tourist destination frequented mainly by those with interest in the wilderness. Leaves crunched beneath my feet as I started my journey.

They were a mosaic of earth tones like brown, red, and orange.

The autumnal graveyard was a welcoming carpet to all or any those entering this ancient forest.

The scent of October echoed throughout the woodlands, an equivalent we all smelled when jumping in piles of raked leaves at the sting of our parent's yard.

There was something solemn that time of year.

Nature was tearing herself down to organize for the approaching cold.

It was the death before rebirth.

Trees around me were showcasing a shocking display of colours.

The pines were unchanged and constant, wafting a subtle mint scent into the air.

As I walked along, I used to be struck by all of the various sorts of foliage that came together to make that scene.

It was even more impressive than I had imagined while sitting in my bed in the dark.

The sky was deliciously overcast on the day of my hike.

A drizzle received the land and me.

I pulled my coat more tightly around myself in an attempt to combat the coolness.

It was only getting to get colder as I started my ascent into the trees.

The raindrops seemed like tiny taps against the leafy forest floor.

It was the foremost effective noise.

I couldn't help but feel utterly asleep as I listened to the natural chorus.

I was utterly free from the burden of acting civilly or fitting in.

The wind and drizzle were the sole movements around me.

There was no change in the landscape for an extended while.

I just kept walking along, losing myself in the gentle noises all around me.

I would occasionally encounter quartz in the ground; it might catch my attention.

The rock's attractive design had always fascinated me.

Even when the sides were worn by the hands of your time, the straight lines of the formation were so unusual.

I had nothing else planned thereon day, so I used to be thoroughly liberal to stop and admire every detail of my hike.

I believe it's essential to allow yourself time to enjoy the wildlife.

It is the environment that birthed us.

I could hear various birds chirping softly as I neared the bottom of the mountain.

I was finally getting to be experiencing the more psychically taxing leg of my adventure.

Nothing beats the scenery on a hike like that.

The exhilaration that I felt brought me intimately to the brink of nature.

I was forging a bond through this trip that might allow me to go to these scenes whenever I needed to call up a peaceful place.

It became a vacation in my head.

A brook was steady, babbling ahead on the trail.

I was going to need to cross it. Hopefully, it would be shallow and unthreatening.

I allowed myself to mentally fall back to the sound of soft, rushing water.

I imagine my troubled thoughts being cleansed; tension washed away.

I had been walking along among the gorgeous damp trees, but the tiny brook marked the gateway to a clearing.

I knew from experience that I used to be getting to be walking alongside a river soon.

I loved the way the rapids spun up foam and raced over rocks and tree roots alike.

The clearing was a small field of patchy grass that allowed me to glimpse the turbulence above me for the primary time in a while.

Massive storm clouds hung above my head.

They were expansive and looked to be made from pale smoke rolling into a deep slate sky.

It had only drizzled thus far, but the weather looked angry.

Most people would rotate, but I used to be excited to ascertain the forest in the throes of a storm.

I passed the clearing and trekked alongside the river.

The water always seemed to be more excitable on the sting of an excellent rain.

I was witnessing a moving painting.

The smooth liquid forming an overflow of the massive boulders stuck in the path was hypnotizing.

My shoes began to make a squishing sound upon the damp leaves as I walked.

It was past the river that I started to encounter the winding parts of my trail.

Fragmented rock jutted from the side of the mountain in jagged pieces.

He might find water running down most of these formations.

Nature must be a master sculptor.

The hours were passing as my journey continued.

I had just exited the thick forest when daylight began to wane.

I was treated to an ethereal deem. I made my way toward the rocky peak of the mountain.

As I looked out over the ridge, I could see where the jagged range melted into the woodlands and jutted back out of the world.

These images had echoed through my thoughts nightly before I made that trip.

I was caught breathless by the great big thing about the protruding angles that dipped into the valley below.

The colours of autumn are stunning.

The landscape looks like one giant earthy ember under the dreary fading light.

The terrain around me was becoming slick with the newly fallen snow.

There was something utterly peaceful about being allowed to witness life from this attitude.

There were no sounds aside from those from the sunshine snowfall.

The world seemed to be entirely still.

I was in with the clouds, ready to touch a few as they passed around me.

I was determined to reach the top before nightfall.

The land around me had turned to pure snow.

I was finding it difficult to believe that it had ever been anything.

The evening was my favourite time of day.

I am crazy with shadows and fading visibility.

I finally reached the height and stood silently searching at the vista before me.

Clouds and large mountains stretched as far as I could see.

The weather had cleared up, allowing me to cherish the icy scene before me.

The snow began to sparkle as I moved my eyes to survey it.

The air was thin and cold. I used to be utterly alone, quiet, still, and asleep.

That was the instant that I had been preparing for.

Every single time I closed my eyes in the dark, I could see myself standing there at the top.

It felt like I used to be always meant to measure that moment.

I descended the mountain some to line up my tent in a part that was rockier than snow-covered.

There was a full-of-the-moon watching over me as I cooked my meal ahead of a crackling fire.

The light and heat were a pleasing contrast to my current environment.

I looked at the cosmos with gratitude for my journey.

I was in awe of the sweetness before me.

I could see the snowy peak bathed in the pale glow of moonlight.

I could have lived in this moment for the remainder of my days.

Allowing the distractions to slide away can enable us to a far better check out ourselves, and it doesn't hurt to possess a view while you're doing all of this.

The following day, I woke myself up before sunrise.

I made coffee and another fire to take a seat and watch the day begin.

It was breathtaking.

The sherbet lights illuminated the sky and painted the rocky landscape with neon hues.

I had never felt so alive as I did at that moment while witnessing the beauty that nature has got to offer.

Midnight Ocean

Clara clapped her hands excitedly. "Tonight's another one, right, Mom?"

She held the massive book in her tiny hands, positively shaking with enthusiasm as Jenny sat on the bed.

"Which one is it tonight?"

Jenny took the book and opened it to a different chapter. The painting showed a "2" in the shape of a seahorse.

Behind it had been a colourful reef standing over a seabed: reds and oranges and blues and greens, bright fish swimming among swaying seaweeds, an eel was winding its way in and out of the reef, crab crawling across the silt.

As they looked, bubbled streamed out of some hidden opening in the reef, and the crab darted to safety because the eel came trying to find it.

A school of fish obscured the view before disappearing in a rush of bubbles.

"Yes, baby, this is often one of my favorites, too. Did I ever tell you that time I need to swim with the dolphins?" "You did? You actually did?"

"I did it! But this is often your story now." Jenny smiled and tapped the image shown in the background, a pod of dolphins playfully darting through the water.

"See? I feel that one kind of looks like you...."

* * *

Kylie walked along the beach.

The sound of gulls crying in the air overhead greeted her, mingled with the waves' sibilant lap upon the shore.

White sand stretched before her in a seemingly endless squiggle, nobody but the seagulls to stay her company.

She breathed in deeply, smelling the salt in the air, closing her eyes, remembering how she used to run barefoot upon the beach as a toddler.

The sand still felt even as warm and comforting to her toes now because it did then.

She knelt and brushed her fingertips through the sand, picked some up, and let it slide through her fingers.

The sun shone brightly upon the gleaming waves.

Kylie approached the water's edge, foaming because it lazily crawled ashore then slipped back again.

She remembered that she had a lover here when she was a child, one of the various dolphins that sometimes swam near the beach.

They jumped, flipped, and spun merrily, and she always wanted to be out there with them.

Once, she swore, the dolphins let her swim with them, but in fact, her parents had never believed her.

No one had, but Kylie knew the dolphins were her friends.

They let her be one of them for a little while.

Now that she had moved back home, Kylie wanted to swim with the dolphins again, but they appeared to be gone.

She had come to the beach hoping to ascertain them, but she was primarily alone this morning.

Well, Kylie could make the foremost of it. She laid down in the sand on her back and waved her arms and legs to make a sand angel or a fish, she thought, as she checked it out.

No, now it looked more sort of a dolphin. Yes, that was it, a dolphin splashing happily amid the waves.

The imprint was so lifelike she could nearly hear the high-pitched cries of the dolphins.

Wait, it had been them! Kylie turned happily bent the Ocean and saw the silvery creatures flipping and rolling as they breached the waves and gleefully plunged backtrack again.

She called and waved her hands. One of the dolphins appeared to notice her, and it swam closer to shore, gracefully diving from wave to wave.

"Hello, my friend!" cried Kylie, wading out into the water.

"Hello, my friend!" said the dolphin, lifting its head above the water.

"How you've grown! I didn't recognize you!"

"I could always remember you," Kylie said, beaming. "The star-marks on your fin and your voice are forever in my memory!"

"You are gone for several years, but we are here still, and that we swim from sunrise to moonset! Will you swim with us again?"

Kylie laughed joyously, and for a flash, she had forgotten about the intervening years.

"Yes! I wish to, more than anything does! I want to recapture how it was to swim in your world!"

"Then accompany me," said the dolphin, and he turned and dove into the waves.

Kylie followed, and shortly she found that she swam not as people do, but with fin, fluke, and amazing grace.

She was swimming like a dolphin, and together they raced through the water with the sound of sloshing and thundering underwater pressure.

The other dolphins welcomed them back, knowing an old flame had rejoined them.

Kylie was now in a dream come true; she was a dolphin, and they swam alongside dolphin's people.

The pod raced away, soon leaving the shore behind and flying through the water far bent sea.

Above them, the seabirds circled, but they were in their domain, and this world belonged to dolphins. This morning, it had been Kylie's, as well.

Sunbeams shone like blades down from the surface. The dolphins frolicked amid the golden shafts of sunshine, dancing together through the morning.

A warm wind tangy with salt whipped the surface of the waves. A faculty of brightly coloured fish scattered because the dolphins approached.

Some chased them, their clicks and high-pitched cries signalling hunger and the thrill of the chase to the remainder of the pod.

Others allow them to go; they were too busy, they said, having fun chasing each other and tasting the morning in the water.

As the sun moved through the sky, the dolphins swam a bit lower.

They loved playing among the reefs shortly from the shore, where He found the original magical colours.

Coral of burnt red and sunny orange nestled amid rocks and rolling hills of silt.

Some dolphins went down and kicked up clouds of silt with their tails, then played hide and seek with one another among the clouds.

Still, others were interested in the various things that inhabited the reef.

Dolphin Kylie, for instance, saw an old turtle swimming past. Floating up to the turtle, the dolphin chirped a greeting. "Hello!" said the dolphin, "and where are you going this morning?"

The turtle was old and cagey, but not so old he couldn't answer with one eye fixed on the dolphin.

"Good morning! I'm going home. It's been an extended time now since I walked on the shores of my origin, and that I want

to see them again."

"The land?" said the dolphin. "What a dry place! Give me surf over sand any day!"

"I have known both," said the turtle, "and once I have one, I long for the other. You're young and don't know the other world's decision yet, but with time. you'll wish you'll walk as I do."

"And you'll wish you'll swim as I do! Good day!"

With that, the dolphin sped away, leaving the old turtle to shake his head and continue on his journey.

Dolphin rejoined the pod, whose chatter had grown quite excited in the frenzy of their play.

After all, a warm stream swept its way through the reef and gave it a chance and joy.

A deep, inviting blue surrounded them, an ideal canvas to be painted silver with the dolphins and lots of yellows, greens, reds, purples, and reef colours.

Groups of bubbles erupted from the activity and floated toward the surface, and everyone contained a dream-like Kylie's.

For the dolphins were carriers and friends to many; the Ocean was a dream.

Those that slept ashore came here in their dreams, and people who dreamed in the water embodied the eternal ebb and flow of life here.

"Let's go deeper!" Dolphin cried because the sun sank a bit in the sky.

Alternatively, perhaps it just grew darker the deeper they went.

Out beyond the reef lay a strange and endless land where the ocean bottom fell away in grand canyons, and the plains of silt and seaweed stretched on forever.

There were big shots here, shining like their scales were made from diamonds.

They didn't flee the dolphins; nothing deterred them on their slow cruise for food, but they had little to mention.

The dolphins soon gave abreast of trying to get them to play.

Giant, bulbous jellyfish undulated through the water. A number of them glowed, shimmering light blue and red in hypnotizing waves.

Several dolphins circled them, admiring their translucent bodies and luminous patterns.

The jellyfish said little, a continuing song, a hum, their voices ancient and speaking of older things the young dolphins didn't understand.

Great beds of kelp floated and swayed in the currents.

Eels and gleaming fish floated among the soft green stalks.

Small sharks swam with single-minded determination, trying to find their next meal.

As a rule, the dolphins didn't attempt to play with the sharks because they rarely had anything interesting to mention.

Instead, the dolphins capered around them, drawing their cold envy at the sheer freedom they enjoyed the day in and out.

The kelp had its voice, an extended song of growth.

The song began at heart in the very roots, speaking of the items that crawled in the slime and muck upon the ocean bottom, and because it rose, many other things became entangled in words: currents, fish, and jellyfish, even the light itself.

The tall kelp had seen it everywhere the course of its long life, and it knew the voices of numerous things.

A shadow passed overhead as something obliterates the sunshine filtering in from above.

Long, beautiful notes rang out.

Whales were passing through, majestic giants who roamed from one blue horizon to another.

They shared in the sheer joy of the dolphins, delighting in the embrace of the mother ocean.

But their perspectives were far-reaching, slower, as they swam slowly through the planet.

The dolphins called to them, and the whales called back.

Dolphin swam to at least one, an excellent blue, its eye shining with a few years of experience.

Its body was a reef unto itself, and around it, the very Ocean streamed and rolled royal raiment to suit an old queen.

"Greetings!" cried the dolphin. "You are so vast and beautiful; looking upon you is like looking upon the ocean itself!"

"Thank you!" answered blue. "How I wish I could join your little ones as you frolic above the waves. But this is often my home and that I love her so. Tell me: have you ever heard our songs?"

"I have it! We love them so. We wish we could dive as deep as you!"

"And I wish I could fly as high as you! You're very young. Depth will come to you yet. I'll never fly, but as long as I can dream, I will be able to dream of your people."

"Nay!"-said the dolphin. "For you're the very living dream of all things in the Ocean; your majesty is unrivaled."

Blue smiled, and the whale slowly swam on, her mountainous make vanishing into the gloom.

Dolphin laughed, following her for as long as he could, but soon he had to return to the pod—and Kylie with him.

A cacophony greeted them: the dolphins and their endless chatter, but also the swift hums of faculties of fish, and the tiny, high-pitched voices of the small things that crawled along the ocean bottom.

Before, they stretched on a landscape where seaweeds, kelp, and tiny coral formations wove a tapestry amid the blue depths.

The dolphins were but one group in countless who all joined their music to that of the Ocean.

Over the silty hills, there lay a treasure: a sunken ship, its timbers coated in the muck, its mast still jutting tall, sails filled with holes but still billowing in the current.

It was the dolphins' favourite playground. An old ship, which had lain upon rock bottom for ages and ages, but it had become a neighbourhood of the ocean bottom now.

Little shelled creatures made their homes in the bowels of the sunken ship.

Fish circled its upper decks, finding a way of calm in its long, restful sleep.

One lone octopus floated near a yawning hole in the ship's hull, and the dolphin greeted it courteously.

"Many armed friends! It's long ago I even have seen you!"

"Good afternoon!" sang the octopus, waving its many arms.

The two of them floated into the ship's interior, find it cosiest next to a broken chest filled with gleaming golden coins.

The octopus settled onto the bed of coins and laughed. "This place remains nice and warm. Would you wish to remain here for a nap?"

"I can't," said dolphin, "because we have a long way to get to the islands. But I will be able to peek in on you once we come to this manner."

"Farewell!" The octopus settled onto its golden bed and shortly grew still with peaceful slumber.

Past the sunken ship and its creaking timbers, the Ocean grew wide, darkening slowly because the sun began to sink.

The dolphins swam back for the surface, admiring a deepening orange sky over grey-green waves.

Water splashed and sprayed around them.

The sound was soft and relaxing, the sleepless voice of a dreaming ocean.

Far on the edge of sight, islands like mountains rose out of the horizon.

"That is where we'll go," said the dolphin. "There are many new dreams to await us there. Except for tonight, we'll sleep here."

Night rose to stain the sky's darkest blue, stars shining like pearls.

The dolphins dove beneath the surface of the water, where silvery rays pierced the veil.

All below them was a cloudy blue gloom, but they might still hear the music of the night-fish and the seaweeds.

Somewhere in the distance, the whales' long and sonorous songs drifted to them, lulling the dolphins one by one into sleep.

"Are you glad you came back?" said Dolphin to Kylie, but she sounded asleep, on the beach, lying upon her blanket and dreaming of azure depths and ancient songs.

Dolphin smiled, and he turned to his people, swimming lazy circles around them until eventually he, too, fell into a dream.

And he dreamed of turtles walking upon the white shores, and of Kylie, together with her hair streaming in the breeze.

* * *

Jenny ran her fingers through her daughter's hair. She turned off the sunshine and stopped to look at the aquarium on the vanity near the bed.

A sunken ship held a small chest, spilling golden coins onto the aquarium floor. The tiny octopus had haunted residence there, still as if it had made it from ceramic...

But as Jenny turned to travel, the octopus waved to her, and Jenny waved back.

The Blue Dream Landscape

Before we start this journey downwards into the deepest realms of our subconscious, allow us to take a moment to physically and mentally, and spiritually acclimate ourselves into being with the awareness of our inner sanctum, our internal workings. We'll begin by going to an area of comfort, ideally a bed or a comfortable recliner, and that we will relax our bodies to the furthest extent possible.

Now, close your eyes, staying firmly on your back, together with your arms relaxed at your sides and your legs rested downwards. Take one deep breath in, through your nostrils, counting slowly to four, and one deep breath out, through your nostrils again, counting slowly to four.

Inhale the breath of the spirit and exhale the strain of the day. Now is the time to rest. Become conscious of nothing but the air flowing through your nostrils; envision a gently flowing stream, smooth inhalations and exhalations, your body become weightier and more relaxed with each passing cycle of breath. Allow your thoughts to become completely still as you focus on your core, your coeliac plexus, allowing your ideas to flow outwards past your vision until they escape your being while only holding and retaining the pure awareness of spirit, the holy serenity of the mind and body. Inhale, one, two, three, four, then exhale, one, two, three, four, each breath becoming slower.

One... two... three... four... One... two... three... four... One... two... three... four... One... two... three... four... One... two... three... four... One... two... three... four...

Continue this pattern of breath, expanding, and sink deeper into yourself, becoming a voyeur of your own still, relaxed body, lost in time. Become lost in this experience as you journey further into the trance, and steel yourself against the road we are close to embarking upon. Draw further and further away from your still, lying body and into the realm of imagination, where images grow, the land of dreams that you are close to becoming one with. Erase your mind of all that's in it currently, and prepare the landscape for a new and fresh experience in the farther reaches of reality.

One... two... three... four... inhale... One... two... three... four... exhale... One... two... three... four... inhale... One...two... three... four... exhale...

Now, with your mind, body, and spirit rested, entranced, and fertile, let us start.

You are lying in your bed, flat on your back, your legs straight out, your arms flat at your sides, your pineal eye acknowledged, up into the sky, your two eyes closed, your mouth still and shut, your nostrils flowing in and out with oxygen. There's nothing but darkness, black, still, and solid, with a lightweight, almost invisible vibrating blue glowing through it, as if at the sides of reality, erosion.

You breathe, stupidly, your core expands in and out, giving breath to your being, and with each breath, your body becomes lighter and lighter, until it's so light, you start to lift it from your bed. Through the sheets, through the blankets, up into space, you're in the middle of the room, hovering, up, and up, through the ceiling, through the roof, into the sky. you're so relaxed; you do not think to worry. You're merely experiencing this, this happening. You want to be asleep.

Your eyes are closed, and your face is pointing up, but you'll see everything below and around you. You see the cars in the streets, parked, owners, drivers, and

216

still and asleep inside their houses. Farther away, lights are on, and there are slight rumbles, noise in the quiet of the night. The streetlights are on, and they are glowing, and you feel as if their shines might house numerous, intangible souls, disembodied, as you're now. You float up and up, and with each distance procured, new sights are visible on the periphery. You see the whole skyline, the sides of the town that houses the population of humans, bleeding into the wilderness, over the foothills, into the mountains, where all is dark, pitch dark.

The darkness looks like where you'll find yourself, magnetically drawn; as you go upwards, the lights will dim, becoming farther and farther away, and you'll be dark. Though you'll not stop it if you tried, you'd not want to, for this darkness, sort of a moth to a flame, is what you crave the foremost. In your sleep, you go up, and you have now reached the clouds. The dots comprising the town below you dissolve into this overwhelming grey mist, and you recognize you have transcended one realm into a new one. You'll not reminisce on the city again, not tonight. Up and up, cloud after cloud, sometimes between clouds, and out of them, you see the pitch darkness amid the distant stars. There's nothing around you, immediately, put deep purple darkness and the black-grey clouds. You pass through them and don't know where they end or where they began; somewhere above the town, and now somewhere below space. You reach the sting of the bank of clouds, and opened to you may be a dark purple abyss as far as are often perceived, stretched up to a pitch-black infinite array of space and stars.

You recognize there's a really, very great distance to travel between the clouds you came from and this space, and as you experience transcending through the layers, you become more profound and deeper into the trance you were already in. As you're, you're merely an expanding consciousness, barren of body, totally light, floating up, by the laws of physics, up and up, forever. You're expanding as you allow the atmosphere of the world, and, with the expansion, you're lighter and lighter.

So light, you'll not even exist, and should be this setting, this environment, experiencing itself from every angle. Who were you again? And where did you come from? You're now in space, going up, up, and up. The moon becomes huge, shining pure white in the black of the sky. It glows, and its glow may be a glow that you can feel in your very being, like a fantastic high frequency vibrating through a part of you, whatever you're now, up here, floating, freely, nothing. It is a purifying vibration that translates you into a fresh, total renewal, even on this voyage previously. You have more lost yourself as you go past the moon into a new, even more vast, experienceable, massive, dark, endless and endless abyss.

Whereas before you had fixed points, you'll recognize above you, being the ceiling, the clouds, space, the moon, now there's nothing, nothing but the stars, which are thus far away from you they'll also only exist in your imagination. But, still and effortlessly, you're making your way towards them, ever slowly. Rising, and up, and up, and up, and up, and up, and up, this new being, transmuted by the glow of the moon, so light so on not even exist, transcending all known borders of the human experience, the reality on earth, now in oblivion, and floating, up.

While your eyes are closed the entire time, your perception of sight only occurring in how completely non-physical and barren of the body, now it's as if your whole being has closed its presence, for there's nothing but blackness. Now even the stars are invisible, somehow, for a few reasons, though you recognize they're out there, somewhere. There's only blackness, and, as some time passed, the slowly revealing electrically charged blue beginning from behind the curtain, the undercurrent, erosion at the pitch-blackness, some subtle energy that exists in the space beyond, always there, interconnected, glowing beneath the surface of our reality.

The boundaries of existence are dissolved, as you now realize, this blue is all there's, you're floating up directly in a sea of sentimental electricity, a buzzing, a hum, that vibrates your whole being, the molecules vibrating out into it until they're spread thus far apart they appear to be scattered evenly across the entire universe. This buzzing, humming blue, scuttling about across eternity sort of a swarm of insects, has become you, and it's you as you're floating up past space and into a deep, dark sleep, dreaming of blue.

Eleanor and the Ship

Kai was always so curious and dreadfully restless. She was up before the first hours of dawn, peeping through her window, wondering if adventure would come to her today. During breakfast, as she ate in the cosy kitchen with her mother and father, she would stretch so she could look out the window and see if anything interesting was outside.

Before lunch, she would stand outside the door, peering, searching in the bushes, learning for shiny stones and metals, then frolic in the garden one last time to plan an adventure.

And when it had been time for dinner, her eyes would be heavy, her body exhausted, and her mood down because she didn't find any adventure today.

The following day, she would awaken in the early hours of the morning, unable to get enough sleep, then she would redo the procedure again; the search for adventure.

Today she peered out the window, expecting to find nothing. But, to her surprise, there was something very, very interesting on the lake just behind her house. She rubbed her eyes to make sure she wasn't dreaming.

There was a ship on the lake! And it was massive! Kai rushed to see it in excitement when their mother called her.

"Kaina Mary Roosevelt!" Mother called, and Kai cringed.

When mother used her full name, Kai knew there was trouble in sight.

"Yes, mother," Kai said, putting on her brightest smile.

"Where do you think you're going?" Mother asked, standing with her hands on her hips.

"Ummm...to the...you see there is a ship...you see and that I just... I just want to get a glimpse, nothing much, just a glimpse, and I will be right back," Kai said, smiling.

"Take a look at yourself," mother said; she didn't look happy.

Kai slowly looked down at her clothes; she was still wearing her nightgown, she was also barefoot, and when she slipped a hand through her hair, she realized it was like a raven's nest.

Kai grimaced and bowed her head.

"And I think I do not need to mention the state of your room, do I?" Mother asked, and at this point, she wore an amused smile.

Kai didn't even wait for a reply; instead, she rushed down to her room.

When she gets to her room, she collapsed on her bed with a sigh and groan, then she remembered the ship, and she jumped up and headed to her window so she could get a nice look at it. It had been beautiful, and it glowed in the early morning sun because the sun rays bounced off its body.

Kai's smile returned fully, and she hurried to clean her room.

She made her bed, made sure the sheets were straightened out and placed the pillows correctly.

Next, she checked out the walls in her room that He painted a bright purple, and she adjusted all the image frames on them, and Kaina had many picture frames on these walls. She was pleased with every single picture, and she changed them carefully.

Next, she grabbed a brush and swept her floor. The dust rose from it had been tremendous. Kaina was shocked at how dusty her floor was.

Her mother came and stood beside her just outside the room, and they both watched how dust covered her room.

"Yes... I do know it is a disaster. Now start working, Kaina's Mother said as she continued walking down the corridor; then she walked down the steps, and Kaina watched her descend.

She looked at the dusty floor and cringed.

How would she get to the ship if she had to clean up this mess?

She stretched and stood on tiptoes to see the ship from above the clouds of dust in her room.

It was still there!

Next, she hurried, and found a mop and bucket, and cleaned the ground.

She got a stool and cleaned all the windows; then, she washed her closet and her reading table, which was at the far end of the space by the second window in her room.

Kaina cleaned and cleaned for the next few hours till her room sparkled and smelled like roses. She stepped into the toilet and washed it till she could see her reflection in the now shiny tiles.

She gave a smile of satisfaction and looked at the gorgeous room, sparkling due to all of the efforts she had put in today.

Never had she worked so hard?

She looked out the window and blew a kiss at the ship by the lake.

"Hold on adventure; I'm coming for you," Kaina said gladly, and she hurried to tidy away all of the cleaning supplies and have her bath.

*****

The only sounds in the room were the clock's ticking and the silent rhythm of Kaina's breath as she slept. The adventurous slave was utterly exhausted from all the diligence she had put in today and slept soundly.

225

Her breath formed a timeless rhythm with the sound of the clock. The clean and quiet room felt, looked, and smelt sort of a haven.

The bed looked crispy clean, the floors glittered, and one could see their reflection on them, the windows were bright and clean, and the moon shined brightly into the room. One could see the ship on the lake.

The second window's reading table was neatly arranged with roses in a vase, placed daintily thereon. The bedroom held the wonderful scent of the roses.

And Kai slept soundly.

*****

The following day Kai awakened utterly astounded. How had she forgotten about the ship! She stared in confusion at the bed and her room.

She must have slept off after cleaning the bedroom, but why had nobody woken her up.

She stretched and yawned as she stood up from her bed and headed straight to the toilet. She stumbled a bit and squeezed her eyes open and shut again to get rid of the sleep and tiredness.

She was stiff; how long had she slept?

She checked the clock just by the restroom door.

It was 7 am!

Had she slept for 14 hours?

Kai shook her head; wow, she must have been more exhausted than she had thought. She squinted at the sun and saw the ship. Excitement pulsed in her veins, and she hurried to have her bath.

She made sure her room was clean; then, she dressed up and headed down the steps. When Kai got downstairs, she checked the mirror in the hallway before getting into the living room to mention hello to her mother and father. "Hello-" the words froze on her lips. Her parents were having breakfast with sailors and what seemed like a ship captain. Kai's eyes widened; could it be? It had to be? The ship on the lake?

Kai saw the sailors in her house, real-life sailors in her home.

Mother turned just in time to see her.

"Kai, you're up. Finally, you're awake. You've been asleep for hours," mother said with an endearing smile, and Kaina walked over to give her a hug and a kiss on the cheek, and she did the same for father. "Captain Jack, meet my daughter Kaina Mary Roosevelt," her father said, beaming proudly. Kai was just glad she had brushed her teeth, had her bath, combed her hair, and worn clean clothes before coming downstairs.

"Hello Kaina, it's a pleasure meeting you," the captain said, smiling brightly. He had kind green eyes that had Kaina smiling back at him.

"You can call me Kai; everybody does," Kai said, still smiling.

"Why in fact, these are two of my crewmen, Micheal and Taylor and this is often my son Jackson junior and my daughter DrusKai," said the captain proudly.

Kai noticed a boy and girl who was almost her age seated at the far end of the living room, watching the TV. She had not seen them earlier because she had been so focused on the sailors.

Kai hurried over to say hello. It had been a long time since Kai had seen children of her age come visiting, so seeing these two children made her very glad.

"Hello, nice seeing you," she said as she joined them on the settee to watch the TV with them.

The girl named Drusilla smiled brightly "nice to meet you too. I'm so glad to meet a person my age," DrusKai said, and before Kai could reply, Jackson Junior interrupted saying,

"Yesterday we came to play but your mother said you were sleeping. Does one always sleep for that long?"

Kai laughed, shaking her head. "No, I cleaned my room and was so exhausted and just fell asleep once was finished, "she said"

"It must have been messy," Jackson said smiling, he had green eyes a bit like his father, and they glowed with friendliness and joy.

Kai liked them both already. DrusKai's eyes were more emerald than green, and they glowed with such an incredible intensity that you wanted to look at all of the day; she had fiery red hair and a soft smile that looked angelic. Kai couldn't help but smile back at the divine beauty.

"Would you like to show us your room?" DrusKai asked together with her eyes wide.

Kai nodded eagerly. She had cleaned this room for hours. She would gladly show it off.

So together, all the youngsters raced up the steps, and Kai proudly presented her room to them.

"Wow," said DrusKai, "it's so neat and pretty," she added.

Kai smiled

"It's bright and colorful," Jackson said, and Kai beamed.

"Would you wish to see our room on the ship? It's decorated a bit like our room back home," DrusKai said, smiling. And Kai's heart skipped a beat, a chance to get to the touch, walk, and see that lovely ship up close? Kai would accept it for the world!

She raced after the youngsters, all the way out of the house, and headed straight for the lake.

She heard their laughter behind her as they hurried to catch up together with her.

When Kai finally made it to the lake, she could only stare in awe. The ship was a beauty, a dream, standing with such magnificence and beauty under the glowing sunlight.

"It's beautiful, isn't it?" Jackson whispered beside her, and Kai could only nod. "Come on, let's enter," DrusKai said

Kai couldn't believe she would get to enter the ship.

Together the youngsters walked into the ship, and the crew members working on the boat said hello to Drusilla and Jackson, and the children introduced Kai to all of them, then they said hello to her also.

The crew was amiable and happy as they worked together. Finally, the youngsters need to DrusKai's room, He had fitted it a princess, and it had been clean too! Kaina's eyes widened, "Wow," she said.

"Come let me show you my room," said Jackson, pulling Kai with him, and when she walked into his room, she wasn't any less stunned.

Kai felt so proud to be ready to stand among these two children with clean, beautiful rooms on a ship, knowing she had a clean and lovely bedroom too. She smiled happily; the boat was fantastic!

Suddenly the youngsters' image, the ship, and the rooms began to disappear, and Kaina awakened on her bed, and she stared in confusion at the place around her.

She was meant to get on a ship!

She stared out the window. The ship stood regal and delightful under the sun.

She checked out her room, clean and sparkling, then why was she not on the ship?

She had her bath, cleaned her room, dressed up, and hurried down the steps.

When she gets to the living room, she met her parents, having breakfast with some sailors, a bit like in her dream, and Captain Jack, who she had seen in her dream! She stretched and saw two children, a boy and a woman watching television at the far end of the living room. It had been DrusKai and Jackson!

Mother turned just in time to watch her wake up and said, "Kai you're up. Finally, you awakened. You have been asleep for hours," mother said with an endearing smile, and Kaina walked over to offer her a hug and a kiss on the cheek. She did the same with her father, but now she started to smile.

She had dreamt about today!

And she couldn't wait for the journey to start.

Twilight

Stephanie's apartment was tiny.

Sometimes it felt like living inside a microwave.

She was sad about the air conditioning going out.

How did people live like this?

She thought, slamming her arm into a pillow on the sofa.

She opened every window in the house, taking some moment to admire the town.

The neon lights were a source of inspiration for the girl.

She loved almost everything about living in the city, aside from her tiny abode.

Stephanie didn't need space, such a lot, because of the ability to inhale the summer.

The youthful woman relinquished of her night in.

Her closest friend Louis lived in the apartment across the hall.

She knocked on his door in hopes of finding him that night.

Louis opened the door, looking wild as if he had been asleep.

He was also soaked through with sweat.

His thick dark hair was rebelling against his usual desire for order.

"I was so on the brink of sleep. Do you understand how irritable it's to sleep in this heat?" He mumbled.

"Well, there's no use now. Better go gets changed and follow me. I can't sit therein sauna." Stephanie said. "No. You do not ruin my rest then demand that I do as you say. Farewell and good luck." He said as he tried to shut the door.

"I am sorry! It's unbearable. If you choose a brief walk with me, I will be able to buy you food, and that we can both stroll in the night air for a short time."

She said together with her foot wedged in between his door and the frame.

"I am unsure you understand where the warmth is coming from." He said.

"Well, at least it isn't stagnant. I won't complain subsequent time you would like me to accompany you to some horrible avant-garde play." Stephanie said.

"I would really like this in writing before I commit."

"Well, I can handle that while you discover a less wet shirt." She said.

Moments later, the pair were descending the questionable staircase in their complex.

The whole building was cheap.

Louis could have afforded something more substantial, but he saw a particular bohemian charm in the place.

This charm evaporated the moment the temperature rose to ninety.

The night air was much kinder.

People were passing the pair as they went about their errands.

Being outside in the dark does something to ignite one's sense of adventure.

Everything feels possible.

Stephanie and Louis decided they might capitalize upon this drive for adventure by exploring a little.

Now and then, they might pass beneath a streetlight that was flickering, unsteady in its glow.

They trekked over one sidewalk until they ran across a block that seemed considerably alive.

The people were bustling around.

They decided that they might stop at a bit of diner that looked to be getting any traffic.

It was a hole-in-the-wall establishment that looked to be crammed with others who were unsure where else they ought to be at this hour.

Watching such an abundance of various people interact in the exact location had always been fascinating to Stephanie.

She ordered a cheeseburger and sat mindlessly touching the checkered paper that came in a basket together with her meal. Food in the city beats food from anywhere else, she thought.

It was a phenomenally greasy beauty.

The pair continued to their walk with full stomachs.

The night acted as a shadow to intensify the hazy city lights.

One could hear numerous languages and cultures being expressed as they walked along the busy streets.

Thick clouds of smoke hung in the air like spirits.

The friends were approached by a couple of strangers trying to find a lightweight, change, or direction.

Each time they were friendly but dismissive.

It is often dangerous to interact with those you don't know, which is why they traversed the terrain together.

Stephanie was the primary to note a bright multi-coloured neon sign that indicated a fortune teller in the area.

Louis immediately sensed that she was curious about finding the place and commenced to protest.

He wasn't in the least bit curious about giving someone his money to make vague deductions about the type of person he could be.

Stephanie was bent to find the building.

She was sure that it might be a stimulating experience, albeit they weren't ready to obtain any reliable information. She was the type of one that collected memories like these and stored them away.

She would search for any opportunity to tug her stories out, bringing an ideal centre.

The pair walked along the cracked sidewalk beneath a radiant full-of-the-moon.

The smog from the town usually obstructed celestial displays, but Luna's power was too strong.

She lit the way for the buddies so that they could never stray on her watch.

The air that night appeared to fizzle with electricity and possibility.

As they walked, they suddenly became aware that they were being followed.

Stephanie grabbed the arm of her friend, and that they quickened their pace.

She whispered to Louis that they might seek refuge in the next business they found.

Looking back, they both believed that it had been a tactic from Madame Hallow to acquire customers.

They darted into the subsequent dark doorway they found before reading the name on the plaque.

The sign read "Madame Hallow's Fortune Telling Grotto."

It was unusual to ascertain a neon sign advertising a business that wasn't marked from its actual location.

There was an extended and carpeted hallway with several doors on either side.

Wood panelling lined the walls around them.

Louis was ahead, and Stephanie pushed him along.

She was scared of being seen from the front window and interested by the establishment.

A strange elderly lady stepped out from behind one of the doors.

Her skin was weathered by the hands of father time.

She had long white hair that she had braided to at least one side.

The lady wore an extended and tattered purple robe that looked to be made out of velvet.

The pair were stunned by the vision of this stranger.

They both understood that she was probably Madame Hallow.

Her eyes were a brand of untamed that neither of the young adults had encountered before.

She could have been named in a horror movie.

She wordlessly motioned for the buddies to follow her.

Madame Hallow passed several doors in the hallway before descending a flight of stairs. Louis and Stephanie entered the basement behind her.

It was empty apart from a card table that sat in the centre with a couple of chairs lining the perimeter.

He told them to sit down.

Her voice didn't match her face.

It was soft and smooth, like that of a toddler.

The pair joined her at the table, and she took a deep breath.

"What am I able to tell you about your future?" Madame Hallow asked.

"Well, we just stumbled into all this. I'm not even sure we would like our fortune told.

What are your rates?" Stephanie asked.

"I will tell you everything for 50. You came to find me for a reason. Who goes first?" Madame Hallow said.

"I guess I will," Louis said hesitantly. The lady grabbed his hands and commenced to rub her thumb along his knuckles. "Let me concentrate. There's something that the spirits want me to inform you.

There is a striking orange fish in your future.

You must follow it down the trail that it shows you." She said.

The lady went on about more personal business that appeared to be accurate educated guesses.

Stephanie watched uncomfortably from her friend's side.

She was going next.

She sat before the older woman, shaking just a bit from her nerves.

She held out a hand to the lady who took it and closed her eyes again.

"You also will follow this fish. It is a journey 2 of you meant to take together.

You must remain close to each other," The lady said.

She didn't even continue Stephanie's reading; she released her hand.

She flipped over her hand as if to request the cash that she was owed.

The pair split the cost between them and then quickly left the basement through a door to an alley in the back.

She told them that those miscreants wouldn't bother them again, but they had never mentioned being followed.

The pair walked back to their complex beneath the dizzying city streetlights and neon signs.

They laughed at one another occasionally about the experience they had had. Stephanie was right; it would bring an excellent story at some point — Expensive but still fascinating.

A week passed before they talked about it again.

He frantically knocked louis on Stephanie's door.

She opened it with a smile on her face as he wasn't usually this excited.

"There exists a large apartment house opening its doors in two weeks.

We can submit our applications now!

We need to hurry, though, because it's expected to be complete super quickly." Louis said.

"My credit isn't nice, so I'm unsure that it's even worth trying. Besides, how much would this cost?" Stephanie asked.

"Just as much as we are paying now. We could get a two-bedroom and it's such a lot larger. It's perfect!" Louis said.

"That sounds amazing, but again bad credit," Stephanie said.

"That is the best part! I feel fate is on our side." He said.

"Why does one say that?" She asked.

"Listen, the name of the place is named Koi Cove." He said with a smile on his face.

Dawn of the Moon

Once upon a time, a person and a lady lived in a remote place, far away from anything. His name was MOON, and Ela was her name.

MOON had white skin, and Ela was brown. It didn't matter initially, but over time there would be tiny little cracks, first in minor ways, then in ways they couldn't hide anymore.

MOON first saw Ela in a room crammed with smoke and decided he wanted her; he tried to understand the taste of her brown skin, he tried to run his hands over her ample body's soft curves. Ela never believed him. She didn't think much about fairy tales or herself or any of it. MOON chased her and chased her; then, she let him take her to dine because she was starving.

At her place, Ela let him have a drink because she was lonely. She let him touch her as she was particular quite hungry. She lay with him and enjoyed his body's meat against her, how sweetly his rough hands kissed her; he brushed her shoulder together with his lips. MOON gave her joy, giving him pleasure, and then, lying next to her, breathing heavily. Ela was grateful.

She ordered him to travel. He did but promised to return, despite her protests.

MOON sent Ela a gorgeous bouquet of scented wildflowers. She called to thank him, and please don't do this again, but she placed the flowers in her front room on the cocktail table and smiled at them constantly. He kept calling, and sometimes she answered, and they spoke about all types of things. MOON continued in his search, and Ela eventually relented and joined him for more dinners; sometimes, they had drinks, and sometimes they saw moving pictures, and she still let him spend the night. Indeed, Ela had forgotten that there was ever a time she wouldn't want MOON around.

The guy looked so different. Ela always thought he was too distinctive. MOON worked together with his hands and had never been far away from something outside the distant area's walls. He learned about the stars and the Sun's location. In the heart of the deep woods, he knew about hidden waterfalls, and he showed them to her, letting her drink the cold, clean water from his rough, calloused hands. Ela's played together with her mind and her heart sometimes. She was familiar with words and spent her days writing books. She spoke various languages and had travelled through oceans to countries and even farther. She longed to be closer to places where she could see bright lights and busy streets and where she could see someone looking like her once in a while. Yet Ela had to do employment and complete studies. She was biding her time. MOON and Ela knew nothing similar to things, but he knew the way to kiss her and the way to press her lips to her neck and the way to carry her as she slept, and if the moments shared between them were all that mattered, they might probably have found a cheerful ever after.

Other things mattered, however. MOON had an evil mother who lived high on a hill in a grand home. She maintained an influential garden and enjoyed welcoming guests to a spacious front room lined with big and imposing furniture.

Quite she grinned, the evil mum scowled. The wicked mother believed her son to be a king and wanted nothing but the best for her eldest child. She didn't think Ela was ok, and she let this be known everywhere on the planet. Ela gave gifts and type words to the MOON's evil mum. She thanked her, please, and she offered to scrub the dishes when invited to dinner. The wicked mother who didn't want MOON to like a lady with such different skin couldn't sway any of her movements. It was something of a scandal, she said. Believe the name of his son, she said. Eventually, Ela started heading up Capitol Hill to the grand home. She and MOON pretended it didn't interest the evil mum. Her disappointment, they told themselves, was an unfortunate fact. We resisted harsh words and blunt thinking. They believed that nothing could get in the way of their happiness and ever after. However, when there was a lot to celebrate on festival days, Ela still found herself alone and waiting while MOON paid his respects and was feasting together with her kin. Ela wanted MOON to settle on in those lonely moments, but she didn't dare inquire; she couldn't bear thinking he wouldn't want her.

A day came when Ela learned that she was carrying the MOON's child. It had been a blessing, which was unexpected but welcome. He said his heart was so whole it ached when she told MOON. He offered his hand at marriage and his side, an area in his kingdom. Ela said to him that they'd wait and see. It had been she who wanted to mention yes. Both began to organize for a future, and once they saw the doctor and heard their unborn child's pounding heart, they checked out one another and located that they had one thing to share— love. Their happiness so blinded MOON and Ela that they shared their excellent news with MOON's wicked mother, who, when she learned the information of a new heir to the dominion, a bastard heir, she narrowed her eyes into dark, hard slits. She said no such child would ever be remembered or accepted by anyone under her rule, a toddler from two dreadfully different worlds. Ela put her hands to her stomach and tried to guard her precious unborn child against words of such poison. Ela was exiled from her home by the evil mother, and MOON stood by and said nothing, torn between his mother and would-be wife. Ela was trying to seek out how to redeem his silence. She never will forget.

It happened on a mean day filled with exceptional moments, each day when MOON painted the nursery for the infant, a soft shade of pink that might be a woman called Emma. He stood in the room admiring his work, picturing his wife holding their child on the brink of the massive window, maybe looking up at the stars. Ela stood in the kitchen, preparing a superb meal for her man, humming her son, sure of her happiness. She was overwhelmed by a sudden grievous pain in her womb. It had been such a sharp and precise pain that she couldn't make one sound. Ela recalled the last moment was dropping to her knees and saying, "I can't bear to lose this." MOON found her on the ground, bleeding painfully, breathing shallowly after the smell of burning meat filled her room. Everyone mourned the child's loss, but rather than breaking them apart; their grief made them love each other fiercer and fiercer.

When she completed her studies, Ela told MOON that she had to go away from the distant location, distant from everything. She had been offered a task she had been planning her whole life for. She was living with too many reminders of what should are had been too hard. She didn't raise children in a position where their people might still treat them as more hers than his. He told MOON he understood. He said they'll find how to like one another over an unlikely distance. She praised him. She believed in her happiness.

On the eve of her departure, MOON sat on a wooden pier beside Ela. They gazed out on waters illuminated by the stars, their heads dizzy with wine. He asked a lady about the foremost beautiful things she'd ever heard a person say. He presented her with a hoop, a gorgeous pear-shaped diamond. He was trying to manoeuvre the ring on her finger, but it didn't suit. Ela, nervously crying, said it had been a nasty omen. MOON had said they'd repair the bell. He said it had been just a fact, and it didn't matter what specifics were. He said, yes, take this bell, yes sleep in my kingdom here, with me. Ela stared at the exquisite ring and wondered how she'd never shared her love for him. He talked about how he made her forget all the tragedies that had befallen her before he loved her. She tried to prevent it but wept and felt her heart falling apart.

MOON thought the tears indicated that she said yes. Ela handed the ring to MOON, her hands trembling. She said I couldn't stay; I can't believe you were asking. She told me you recognize me not; the specifics matter. She said if you leave this place with me, you ought to have asked. MOON said he never understood other life types. These were his people, he said, and this was his land. He said he'd spend his life making her love the way he did that land, that his family would grow to embrace her. He became furious; she said it had been his; he said he would never let her go. Ela hugged her stomach and recalled the kid growing up there once and how her loss so closely tied them together. They sat in silence together, the night air cooling between. He knew a long time ago that he was right about the fairy tales.

Building Confidence and Becoming Happier

Some situations can cause you to feel "less-than" and burden you with beliefs that you are incapable of doing or having what you would like. It's important to remember that it's not uncommon to wonder how to be more confident in yourself.

It is also essential that you learn how to tap into your inner strength on those days once you don't feel confident because your confidence affects your performance in any area of life. Likewise, your account affects your confidence. The downside to experiencing low self-esteem can present negative emotions and limiting beliefs, which will be easily remedied by applying mindfulness-based lifestyle practices like meditation. There are ways in which you'll build your confidence and be happier through mindfulness; they include;

1. Learning the way to Meditate

There is no "right" way to meditate.

That being said, basic mindfulness meditation is perhaps best due to how easy it's to start. In a nutshell, mindfulness meditation revolves around being "mindful," i.e., specialising in this moment's physical sensations.

Most people still don't know how to meditate. That's okay. Though it brings ease, it is often quite complicated. Many meditation techniques originate from the East, including the Judeo-Christian meditation method, Buddhism, Hinduism, and Taoism. Mindful meditation will assist you in getting in-tuned with everything good that already exists in your world.

Below are a number of the ways to meditate;

1. Sit comfortably in a quiet place.

2. Think about your best quality or something you appreciate about yourself or something you're pleased with, feel positive about yourself, and contemplate this for a short time.

3. Next, identify some positive goals for yourself. These could be: 'I would like to be happy,' or 'I want to be healthy.' Recite whatever phrase comes from your

heart and has the most meaningful to you. Repeat this phrase a couple of times.

4. Once you begin feeling the positivity that comes from adopting a sort attitude to yourself, you'll then take the great feelings outwards by bringing forth a picture of somebody you're keen on and offering them equivalent wishes you have presented yourself.

5. At the top of the meditation, you'll notice how starting this practice with self-love, then directing that love towards others enhances feelings of kindness, compassion, and connection.

Another way to meditate is to;

1. Find a comfortable place and minimize distractions.

2. Close your eyes and start to take some slow deep breaths, following your inhalation and exhalation, to allow yourself to settle into a peaceful, meditative state.

3. Begin by bringing a real-life situation to mind where you would like to be ready to step into a state of confidence. Maybe it's a conversation you would like to have or a presentation you've been asked to deliver.

Perhaps you've been meaning to ask someone on a date or set a meaningful goal.

4. As you bring this example to mind, create an image, then fire off the previously created anchor. You ought to feel yourself shifting to a spirit of feeling confident. (If not, repeat the anchoring process and test it to make sure it works.)

5. Play out the scenario in your mind in the most positive way you'd most wish to see it unfold. Follow the movie reel through to completion, where you finish with the most favourable outcome. Absorb everything you see, hear, and feel around you. Notice how confident you are and how amazing that feeling is.

6. Once you are ready, open your eyes and write about how the process was for you. Repeat as often as necessary.

2. Build the Habit of Meditating

Meditation isn't something that you can do once or twice and instantly reap all of the benefits.

It would help if you meditated consistently to get better. You'll see a clear difference (in terms of your ability to focus and feeling more confident) after about two weeks but don't expect to meditate today and awaken with superhero-level confidence tomorrow morning.

The most effective way to build the daily habit of meditation is to make it a part of your daily routine. You ought to create a morning routine immediately if you don't have one. Once you're comfortable position, sit in silence with your thoughts for 5-10 minutes, it becomes straightforward to catch yourself getting anxious and overthinking things at the moment. Quickly practice mindfulness, stop the negative self-talk, and switch on your natural confidence!

3. When Anxious Use Mindful Breathing

By learning how to meditate and successfully building the habit of meditation, you'll develop a confidence that will stick with you regardless of what you're doing. You'll be missing out on a tremendous advantage of meditation if you do not consciously apply mindfulness to stressful times in your life.

Imagine that you are in a stressful social situation, like when you notice a cute girl, and you would like to approach the bar. However, rather than saying hello, you get nervous and begin to tense up. You start thinking of a bunch of excuses not to approach her or all the ways you'll screw it up, or perhaps you're sitting at home on your own, over-analyzing something that's on your mind. Maybe it's whether or not you ought to ask for a promotion at work. Or you are thinking about why none of your friends has called you recently.

Either way, you stray in a whirlwind of negative thoughts, become entirely paralyzed, and shit yourself. It is what you ought to do instead, focus on your breathing. It works because once you concentrate fully on breathing (i.e., each inhalation and every exhalation), it's tough to think about anything else simultaneously.

Here may be a quick and straightforward way to put this into practice:

You catch yourself getting lost in negative thoughts.

Sit down on the ground or in a chair and ensure a tall and erect posture. Relax your body (especially your shoulders, neck, and chest)

Set a 5-minute timer on your phone

Begin breathing through your nose. Focus on your breathing (like you're doing a mini-meditation)

Feel the cool air enter your nose (and your belly rise) with each inhalation

Feel the nice and cosy air exit your nose (and your body relax) with each exhalation

Take action (do what you're brooding about or advance and do something else)

This simple practice is like a moment of medication to alleviate stress and eliminate anxiety. It is often more straightforward (and works way quicker) if you're used to meditating on a day today. Once you catch yourself brooding about anything besides your breathing (and you actually will), re-focus on subsequent inhalation.

4. Taking note of music

Another way to exercise mindfulness is by taking note of music that soothes you and even singing along. The genre of song that helps you relax doesn't matter. The mindful way to listen is to consider each note. Maybe even dance along! Music may be an excellent way to release stress.

5. Speaking Your Thoughts

Do you find it hard to focus on the thoughts running through your mind? Does trying to ignore these thoughts while meditating stress you out more?

Instead of fighting the notions in your head, attempt to observe them objectively. Consider creating an audio journal. You'll record yourself in your drive to and from work. Rather than fuming while you're stuck in rush-hour traffic, you'll spend the time relaxing your mind. It's a simple way to process what's happening in your head.

Here are five ways mindfulness can cause you to happier and also enhance your self-confidence:

1. It can assist you in getting out of negative thought loops

Meditation allows you to understand that you don't need to hear the voice inside your head, especially when it's negative, and focus on "bad" things about yourself (e.g., how you look, what people believe you, etc.). It becomes easier to "get in the zone," turn your brain off, and stop negative self-talk by meditating regularly. Whether it's loops of worry, planning into the longer term, replaying events from the past, or 261 trapped in self-judgment -- once we develop the skill of mindfulness and convey this quality of awareness to the working of our mind, we open up an entirely new possibility toward greater happiness. We start to possess the facility to be the master instead of the slave of our minds. Meditating can physically alter your brain to be less anxious and more confident.

2. It can cause you to feel more connected to others

We are social animals that have evolved to be in relationships. To flourish, we'd like to feel related to others. Mindfulness can deepen and enrich our relationships as we bring a top quality of present-moment attention to the people around us.

3. It can connect you to a way of inner contentment

Mindfulness may be a practice that will help us cultivate a habit of inner well-being, which allows us to feel content and well without getting anything from the surface world. It's a rare feeling in this age of consumerism, but it's available to all or any folks at any moment.

4. It can enhance your gratitude.

The practice of mindfulness helps us to hamper, albeit only for a couple of moments, and reconnect with what's happening from moment to moment; this slowing down enables us to note more of what's present in our surroundings and ourselves. As we notice more of what's happening around us and in us, wonder and gratitude can spontaneously emerge, whether it's being more present to the tastes of a home-cooked meal or connecting with something as miraculous and straightforward because the breath -- mindfulness can infuse our lives with gratitude and enhance our appreciation of the everyday things which may so often travel by unnoticed.

5. You spend less time worrying about the longer term

The practise of mindfulness helps to stay the mind focused on this moment, suggesting the reason isn't constantly worrying about the longer term. Research shows that 85% of what people worry about never happens. With the 15% that did happen, 79% of subjects realize that they can handle the problem better than expected.

Conclusion

Once again, thank you for reading – "**Bedtime Stories for Adults**."

There are several ways to make time for yourself when daily stress is taking its toll. But what if there was a simple way to escape somewhere else?

Maybe you can't physically transport yourself to a different time or place, but reading fiction can take your mind out of the physical world for a brief time.

Don't worry if you're not a voracious reader – it only takes six minutes to immerse yourself in a story and reduce your stress levels. On Monday, start your week off in a completely different universe before stepping into the daily grind!

Research has shown that reading fiction reduces stress than listening to music, sipping tea, and taking a walk. Stress levels were shown to be reduced by 68% after reading.

While your brain is engaged in the story, your pulse slows down, and muscles relax. Because there's such a lot of work for your brain to do, reading may be a very effective way to focus your energy and improve your concentration. The act of reading something with a "strong narrative arc" also lasts beyond the time you're reading. Your brain will hold on to the story, supplying you with something to revisit later. If you start reading a new book on Monday, you'll have an entirely new world to float off to all week!

On top of being great for reducing stress, reading also increases your emotional intelligence and empathy as you get inside the story's characters' heads and lives. So, if stress makes you feel a little bit hostile towards people, reading might help you be nicer!

The best part about reading as stress relief is that there's no stress in choosing what to read or when. You'll find a couple of minutes first thing in the morning or at lunchtime.

Take out a book if you're on public transport to work, or make reading the first thing you do once you arrive home. Choose something that you genuinely enjoy which causes you to feel happy and calm. (The newspaper or your social media feed are probably not the best options.)

When you've completed your reading, don't stop there – turn your reading experience into something stimulating.

What did you think of the characters?

Did you discover something you have in common with them?

Would you have done things differently than they did?

What about the story did you relate to or enjoy the most?

Remember, you're reading for pleasure – you won't be tested! This is often merely a fun exercise that allows your creativity to blossom while your body takes a breather.

Choose your adventure. When choosing your reading, ask yourself what genre suits your fancy today. Look through your bookshelf, your local library, or get an e-book from the web over the weekend – and begin reading on Monday!

Find the time and place. You don't always have to drop everything to read a book, but by setting aside a couple of minutes and designating an area to read, it'll be easier to dive into your story.

Focus, focus, focus, don't listen to music, don't read with the TV, and don't read with people around. Make it the only thing you're doing – this is often sometimes.

Don't just stop. After reading, allow a couple more minutes to let what you have read sink in.

The most important thing to note is how you feel when you're done. If you're less stressed, then read for longer!

Printed in Great Britain
by Amazon